2-00 .

Patients Are A Virtue

Practicing Medicine in the

Pennsylvania Amish Country

by Henry S. Wentz, M.D.

with illustrations by Paul H. Ripple, M.D.

Patients Are A Virtue

Practicing Medicine in the Pennsylvania Amish Country

Library of Congress Number: 96-80360

International Standard Book Number: 1-883294-49-5

Printed by
Masthof Press
Route 1, Box 20, Mill Road
Morgantown, PA 19543-9701

TABLE OF CONTENTS

A Section on the Amish

Additional Experiences

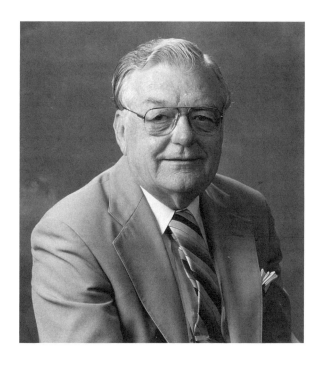

Henry Stauffer Wentz, M.D.

PREFACE

I was born in Leola, Lancaster County, Pennsylvania. My grandfather, Henry M. Stauffer, after whom I was named, had started a coal, lumber and feed business at Leola in 1890. It became a family business, H. M. Stauffer & Sons, in which my father and two uncles were involved. Joseph C. Wentz, my father, was active in the business; and Arline Stauffer Wentz, my mother, was a homemaker. When I was four years old, following the death of my maternal grandmother, I lived in my grandfather's home with my maternal grandfather, my parents and my younger brother, Robert. The family was actively involved in the Methodist Church.

My paternal grandfather, great uncle, uncle and several cousins were physicians. Although I was raised in a business family, I was encouraged at an early age to enter the field of medicine. I enjoyed my work as a physician and am happy I was persuaded by members of my immediate family to follow this career.

During my teen-age years I worked at H. M. Stauffer & Sons; and in the summer of 1942 I was employed at Gilliland Laboratories, now Wyeth-Ayerst, at Marietta, Pennsylvania.

After graduation from Upper Leacock High School in Leola at age 16, I attended Duke University. That is where I met my wife to be, Mary Louise Whitney, from Washington, D.C. We would be married in 1943. Following my graduation from Duke in 1941, I enrolled at Jefferson Medical College in Philadelphia. Because of the pressures of WWII, classes were accelerated. I attended school year-around and was graduated in September 1944. Internships and residencies were reduced to nine months, and I trained for 18 months at the Lancaster (Pennsylvania) General Hospital. After completion of hospital training in 1946, I began service as an Army physician at Fort Sill, Oklahoma until my discharge in 1948 with the rank of Captain, Medical Corps, Army of the United States.

I began the general practice of medicine in Strasburg, Pennsylvania, a village of 2000, in 1948 with my office adjoining my residence. In 1960 I moved to a new location in the same town. I continued to have an office in my home until 1974. At that time three Mennonite physicians and I began a group family practice, Eastbrook Family Health Center, three miles north of Strasburg, just a short distance north of Route 30. I retired from Eastbrook Family Health Center in 1988.

From 1971 to 1974, I assisted Dr. Nikitas Zervanos, Chairman of the Department of Family and Community Medicine, in establishing a family practice residency program at the Lancaster General Hospital. That led to our establishing a model family practice unit in Quarryville, about 12 miles south of Lancaster.

I served short assignments with Care/Medico in Honduras and the Indian Health Service at Standing Rock, North Dakota, and Fort Belknap, Montana. Also, I served in the Dominican Republic with the Christian Medical Society.

Since my retirement, I have been active in researching and recording medical history in the Lancaster County community. I was a member of the Lancaster General Hospital's 100th anniversary committee and chairman of the 150th anniversary committee of the Lancaster City and County Medical Society.

I lived and practiced medicine in Lancaster County my entire adult life except for my education and service in the Army. I have enjoyed a harmonious relationship with the Amish and Mennonite people during my childhood and my medical practice.

These stories are true life experiences during the time of my medical training and practice. I was a family physician in the Strasburg area for 40 years from 1948 to 1988. I was fortunate to begin my medical career after the discovery of the first antibiotic, penicillin, and I saw many monumental advances during my 40 years of practice. I also started my journey when insurance for hospitalization was beginning and witnessed the advances in medical insurance, through government intervention in the health-care arena to the beginning of managed health-care programs.

I saw the growth of specialization in all areas of medical practice, including my own family medicine specialty. My career encompassed the demise of solo physicians practicing out of the home and the establishment of large group practices in sizable medical buildings.

Medicine will never again be practiced as it was in the mid-20th Century, so this collection includes a few stories of human interest. In the early days of my career, hospitals furnished the only ambulances in Lancaster County, and they were manned by an intern, a nurse, a driver and a helper; the era of antibiotics was beginning; indigent patients were treated in large hospital rooms known as wards, and physicians were assigned to the patients. Fees for medical services were the patient's responsibility.

In most of these stories the names of patients have been changed to fictitious names for the purpose of confidentiality and privacy.

It is my hope that the reader may enjoy hearing about the experiences as much as I enjoyed practicing medicine and participating in these adventures.

This book includes a section about practicing medicine among the Amish as well as stories about Mennonites and the rest of us.

I live in Lancaster, Pennsylvania with my wife, Mary. We have two children, William and Louise. Mary and I are members of the Wesley United Methodist Church in Strasburg.

Henry Stauffer Wentz, M.D.

ACKNOWLEDGEMENTS

Many chapters of the book have been illustrated by Paul H. Ripple, M.D. He enjoys art and is well-known for his sketches and illustrations which can be seen in many books and buildings in the Lancaster area. The author is especially appreciative for the sketches that he has contributed to this book.

Dr. Ripple was born and raised in Lancaster, Pennsylvania. After graduation from (Lancaster) McCaskey High School, he graduated from Franklin & Marshall College and University of Pennsylvania Medical School. He interned and had a short residency at the Lancaster General Hospital. Following completion of his military service at the School of Aviation Medicine at Randolph Field, Texas, he took a two-year residency in ophthalmology at Washington University in St. Louis. He practiced ophthalmology in Lancaster, Pennsylvania for 40 years and retired in 1994.

*　　*　　*　　*

The author thanks C. Eugene Moore for his help in editing all the material in this book. He also gave suggestions for titles and the arrangement of the book. Mr. Moore graduated from Auburn University and received a Master's Degree from Florida State University. He retired as Director of Public Relations with Armstrong World Industries, Incorporated, in 1994.

DEDICATION

I wish to dedicate this book to my parents, the late Joseph Clair and Arline Stauffer Wentz, who encouraged my career in medicine and funded my education, and to my wife, Mary, and children, William and Louise, who lived through many of my experiences.

Henry Stauffer Wentz, M.D.

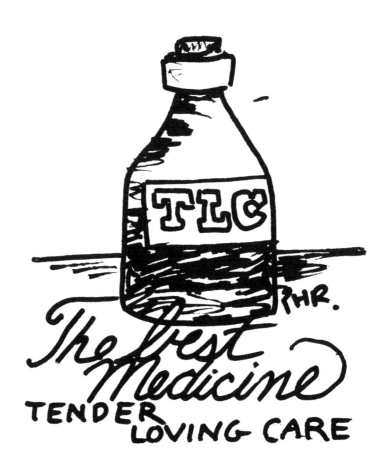

THEY MAKE A DIFFERENCE

The Amish, members of an unusual Christian sect, number about 15,000 children and adults in eastern Lancaster County. Their Amish forefathers emigrated from Switzerland, Alsace and the Palatinate. They believe in adult baptism, pacifism, social separation from the world, obedience to church teaching and shunning (exclusion of errant members from communion).

The Amish have a strong faith in God and their Savior, Jesus Christ, and the Bible. The Old Order Amish are divided into districts usually comprising 25 to 35 families. Each district is headed by a bishop and each may follow rules slightly different from the others. Church services are held in the homes, so an Amish home must be large enough to accommodate the membership of the district. Instead of pews the people sit on benches that are transported to the home by horse and wagon; the women are kept busy preparing the food, as church is an all-day affair. The service is held every other Sunday. Weddings, which take place in the late fall after harvest, and funerals are held in the homes of the district.

Amish families abstain from the ownership, and to a lesser extent the use, of such modern technology as electrical appliances, automobiles and telephones. They use kerosene lamps instead of electric lights, gas stoves instead of electric ranges. For communication they use the mail and person- to-person conversation instead of the telephone. For transportation they prefer horse and carriage to the automobile. They speak German (Pennsylvania Dutch should be Deutsche), though the children learn English in the school. The Amish believe in non-violence and may enter voluntary service in a hospital or other community service instead of serving in the armed forces.

The men and boys wear loose fitting trousers with suspenders. They use hooks and eyes instead of buttons, as they consider buttons too "fancy" or worldly to be acceptable. Their main garb is black, although they may wear bright-colored shirts. They are known for their broad-brimmed straw and dark-colored hats. After marriage the men grow beards. The women wear dresses closed with straight pins instead of zippers or buttons; they wear head coverings (caps) and aprons. They wear black stockings, and the young women may wear bright-colored dresses under their aprons. The bride wears a white apron; this apron is put away after her wedding and not worn again until her death.

They prefer to avoid any formal education of their children after 14 years of age, and in the 1950s they struggled the whole way to the United States Supreme Court to retain this control. The Amish have their own school system, often with their own teachers, and their one-room schools have outhouses.

Amish men believe in making their living off the land, and the large majority are farmers. On their farms they use horses and mules instead of gasoline-powered tractors. Some work in building trades and crafts. The women also work on the farm and in the house. Some women may work as domestic helpers or in small factories.

They have their own insurance. They help each other. The most significant event, which demonstrates working together and helping one another, is a barn raising. If a barn is destroyed by fire, a group will clean up the area while the embers are still hot. Skilled Amish men will plan the new barn, order building materials, and set a date for the construction. The women arrive and help with the preparation of food and drink, and the men come to build the barn. Once the skeleton is in place, the exterior of the building is completed in one day.

As a physician in the community, I had a great opportunity to learn the basic beliefs and truths of the Amish people and to see them live by these concepts.

The stories I tell, which took place in the 1940s through the '70s, portray some of their beliefs and traditions in action. I learned much from my association with these people; and I have always admired their philosophy of life, which is rooted in their religion.

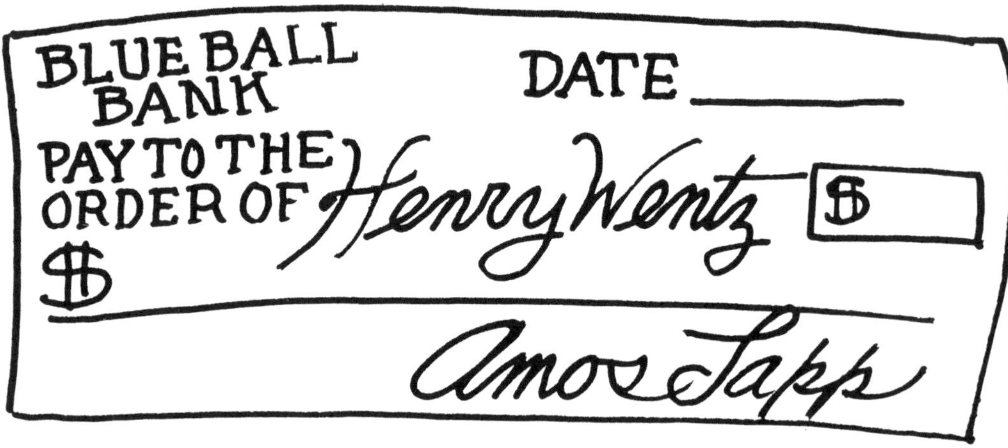
BLUE BALL
BANK
DATE
PAY TO THE
ORDER OF Henry Wentz
$
$
Amos Sapp

A SINCERE TRUST

One of the basic beliefs of the Amish is utmost trust in their fellow man.

I had treated Amos daily for about two weeks for severe pneumonia with daily injections of penicillin and the use of other measures for comfort and eventual cure. (This was in the 1950s, before oral penicillin was effective.) When he came to the office for his last visit for this illness, he offered to pay his bill. At the time I worked alone, with only the part-time services of my wife, so the bill had not been prepared. I said, "I don't have your bill ready at this time, Amos. I will send it to you at the end of the month."

Without any hesitation, he replied, "I have my checkbook with me. I'll give you a signed blank check and you can fill in the amount when you have time."

I remembered that one of my teachers in high school during a lesson on check-writing had instructed her class, "Never sign any check unless you have filled in the amount and the person or company that you are paying."

I said, "But Amos, I could complete that check for any amount I wished."

Amish people call you by your first name. His reply was, "Henry, I trusted you with my life. I don't see why I can't trust you with my money."

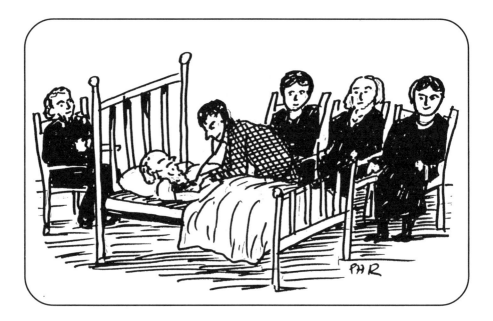

A DIFFICULT TIME

One of the most impressive experiences for a young physician, or any physician, is being called to a Amish home when someone has died.

As I mentioned, the Amish do not have telephones in their homes. But their communication system defies imagination. (Actually, they start gathering when death seems imminent.)

When I receive a call about a death, I usually leave promptly for the home of the deceased. By the time I get there in an automobile, occasionally scores of Amish people may have gathered in the home. The women, dressed in dark clothing, are assembled in one room; and the men, likewise dressed in black, are seated around the perimeter in another room.

As you enter the house, you can hear mutterings. Although most of the conversation is in Pennsylvania Dutch (or, more correctly, Pennsylvania German), you overhear someone saying, "There's the doctor." And you know you are under observation. The same thing occurs as you enter the room in which the men are seated. Usually one or more members of the family will meet you at the door as you enter and lead you through the people. You may see a few familiar faces, which eases the loneliness you feel on such an occasion. You are taken to the room of the deceased, and there you perform your duties. You listen for the heartbeat, which is not present;

you check for signs of breathing, and you examine the eyes for fixed, dilated pupils. Then you assure the family members with you that death has occurred. You complete and sign the death certificate for the funeral director and place it on a table near the deceased. You backtrack through the maze of people, occasionally chatting for a moment with a family member or friend you recognize.

This experience is difficult for family, friends and physician alike.

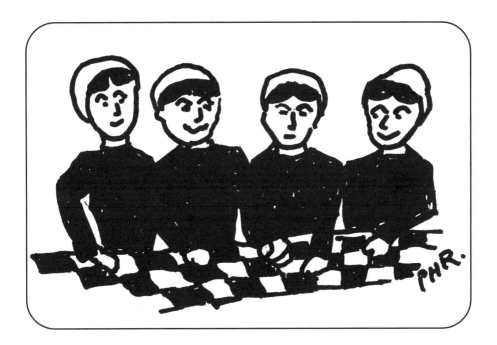

LOVE AND COMPASSION

The Amish people have a wonderful support system, which they have used for centuries. We, whom they call "the English," are gradually beginning to adopt some of their sensible and well-developed customs.

When a death occurs in an Amish family, members of another family who have encountered a similar problem may befriend the bereaved and help them through the ordeal of their sorrow. For example, if an Amish child is killed in a sledding or farm accident, members of a family that have experienced the death of a child in a similar manner may quickly become their "angels of mercy" and empathetically share their compassion. An Amish family that has experienced a death by suicide may be supported emotionally and spiritually by members of a family who have had the same sad event.

Another type of support system is a help particularly for the woman whose husband has recently died. Amish women have quilting bees and the new widows are especially invited and accompanied to these gatherings. The women are sewing quilts while they are performing a useful task of support to their bereaved friend(s). They keep their hands and minds busy as they share their basic beliefs: industry, spiritual and emotional support.

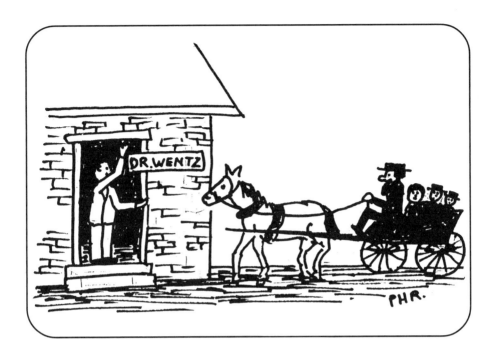

A BETTER UNDERSTANDING

In 1979 three events slammed tourism in Lancaster County: the nuclear accident at Three Mile Island, the shortage of gasoline and the lines of cars waiting to get gas, and several cases of poliomyelitis among the Amish.

The last was caused by a lack of polio vaccine distribution to the Amish people. I was asked to contact some of the Amish bishops, who are quite influential, about the acceptability of polio vaccine among their people. As I discussed the problem with each bishop, I was able to relate incidents of paralysis among some member of their group.

They accepted the concern of the medical community and agreed to recommend polio immunization, provided it was to be carried out under these conditions:

1. Immunizations would be given at places convenient to them, such as at Amish schools. Generally, an Amish school is situated in each Amish neighborhood.

2. Immunizations would be given at appropriate times. Driving a horse and buggy at night can be hazardous. The bishops preferred daylight hours, but at times that would not interfere with the milking time among their dairy farmers.

3. They wouldn't put themselves under any obligation to the state. Mainly, this meant that they did not want the state to pay for the vaccine. They wanted to pay its costs themselves.

The conditions were met. The Amish families cooperated fully. And we were able to administer the polio vaccine to their children.

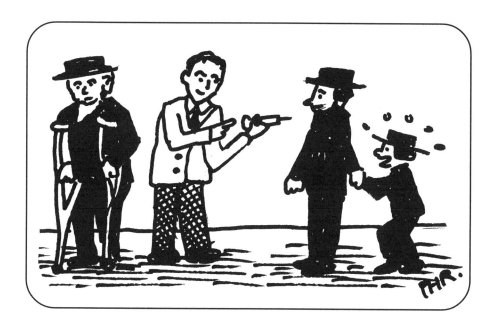

LEARNING IS CONTINUOUS

Ever since I started my medical practice in Strasburg, Pennsylvania in 1948, one of my concerns had been the lack of preventive medicine that I was able to provide for my Amish patients. Women didn't start their prenatal care till late in pregnancy, some parents refused immunizations for their children and neglected well-baby examinations after their children were born.

After a few years, I realized that if I placed too much pressure on these people, they would go elsewhere for their medical care. I began to write down the times I discussed preventive care with them; after two times, or at most three, I would not again mention immunizations or other types of preventive medicine. Sometimes I was bothered by my inability to change their behavior in health care. (You must understand that I am generalizing. Many Amish families accept preventive medicine very well.)

During a portion of my time as a teacher at the Lancaster General Hospital in family medicine, I was fortunate to have with me an Amish man, who was a resident physician in training. He was from a neighboring state, Ohio. Although he was of the Amish faith, he was not a member of the Old Order Amish. He drove an automobile, dressed similarly to the rest of us and had received higher education. He became a member of the health care team at the Model Family Practice Unit of the Southern Lancaster County Health Center in Quarryville. I marveled at his ability to convince his Amish patients—and many Amish families asked for him—to receive immunizations for their children..

One day I asked him, "How do you achieve so much success in providing immunizations for the children of your Amish families?"

He replied, "I explain to them about the dangers of lock-jaw, as a result of injuries, especially working among farm animals. I remind them of some Amish person, probably an acquaintance, who has died of tetanus. Most of them know 'Lame John,' as you and I do. I tell them that they can prevent that type of lameness in their children, if they allow me to administer polio vaccine. The large majority of them accept the idea of immunization when it's explained this way."

That day I gained an important insight. From then on I applied this new method of informing my Amish families about immunizations, and I was amazed at their acceptance of the concept. The Amish may not have much formal education, but they are not ignorant. I became an effective physician when I began expressing the needs of preventive medicine in language that they could understand.

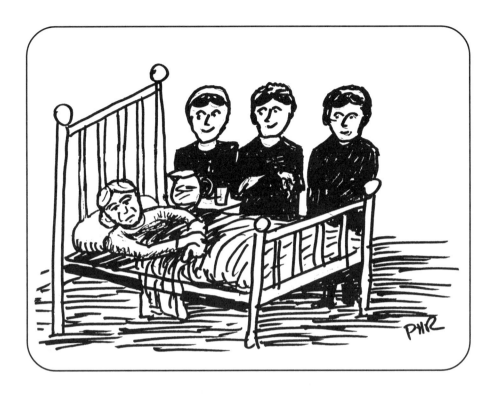

CARING

Ruth, an elderly Amish woman had terminal cancer. She had had surgery and, later, radiation treatments. No further therapeutic measures were indicated for her problem. Her condition was painful. She had three adult daughters living at home. I visited the home and talked to Ruth, who was aware of her condition and unpromising outlook.

Ruth said, "Rachel and Leah and Miriam take such good care of me. I couldn't ask for anything more."

"Are they able to keep you comfortable? Do you have much pain?"

"Pretty comfortable. They try."

"If you let us know when you're in pain, I think we should be able to give you medicine to keep you comfortable."

"I'm satisfied. A little pain never hurt anybody."

"Have all of us explained your problem to you satisfactorily?"

"Oh yes, I know I have cancer. I don't have much longer to live, but we'll make the most of it. You don't need to bother yourself to come down here often. The girls have been taking good care of me. You don't care if they call you or stop in the office once in a while, do you?"

"No, I'll help all I can."

"Thanks for your help."

The three daughters followed me out of the house. Standing beside my car, Rachel said, "We want to take good care of Mother and keep her as comfortable as possible. We have talked it over and don't want you coming down regularly. We will call when we need help or aren't sure what to do. How is she? What can we expect?"

"She is very sick. She will be uncomfortable unless you give her the pain medicine and sedation regularly. Make your main goal to keep her comfortable. Call me when you need me. If you want more medicine, send someone to the office. All of you are doing a magnificent job. Your mother is fortunate to have three loving and compassionate daughters."

"Thank you, Henry."

I left medicine for them to administer to their mother and once again went over the instructions I had given them about caring for her physical needs.

Just before I drove away, I said again. "Call me when you need me."

Sometimes they would call from a neighbor's house about a question they had. Sometimes one of the daughters passing the office would stop in to talk or get more medication. Occasionally over the next several months they would ask me to see their mother. She received wonderful physical care as well as comfort and loving attention.

When at last she died, they seemed satisfied and happy that they had been able to care for her at home and in the manner they desired, without undue intervention by me or other medical personnel.

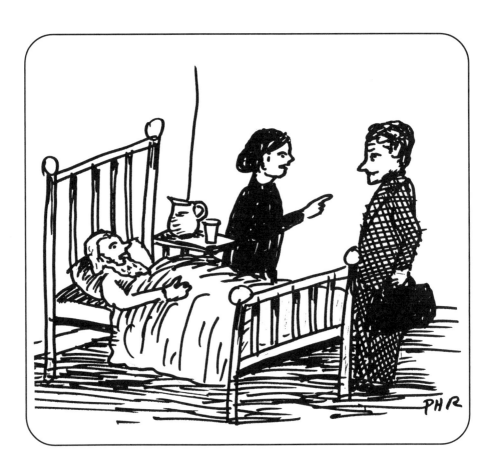

DYING IS A PART OF LIFE

In many instances, death seems to be accepted as a part of life by the Amish people. As a result, many of them don't cherish modern devices or sometimes even hospitalization as a means of prolonging life.

For some years I had been seeing an Amish man, Jacob, for heart disease with disturbances in cardiac rhythm and other problems. His condition was well-controlled, and he had been leading a productive life for many years. In his late 70s he began to have more serious problems, but he and his wife preferred that he stay at home and live with any necessary limitations. About once a month I made it a practice to stop at his home to check on his condition and make any changes in his treatment that seemed appropriate.

Over the past year, Jacob had been failing. Now he was confined to a chair and bed existence. One day as I stopped by on a regular visit, his wife, Mary, met me at the door. She said, "Oh, you didn't come to see Jacob, did you?"

"Yes, I'm due to see him again."

"He isn't doing well at all. I wish you wouldn't bother him."

I looked past her into the parlor where Mary had set up a bed for Jacob. The instant I saw him, I could tell he was having serious problems. I sat down on the sofa with Mary at quite a distance from Jacob, and quietly asked her, "How long has he been this way?"

"Several days."

"What are you doing for him?"

"Keeping him comfortable. I change him when he is wet or messed and give him water or juice if he wants something. His condition is not good, I think."

"No, it isn't. How do you feel about it?"

"I am prepared. The Lord will take care of him and me. I don't want him to go to the hospital. I want you to let him stay at home. You go now. I will call you when I need you."

"Are you getting your rest? Can I help you in some way?"

"No, I don't need anything. There will be plenty of time for rest later."

Jacob had stirred during our discussion. When I was satisfied that she understood and that they had made their decisions, I arose to leave. As I left I said, "Mary, when you need me or want me, call."

She responded, "Thank you for not disturbing him. I will let you know."

A few days later I received a call to go to Jacob's home. The end had come peacefully and gently. He and Mary had spent their last days together as they had wished.

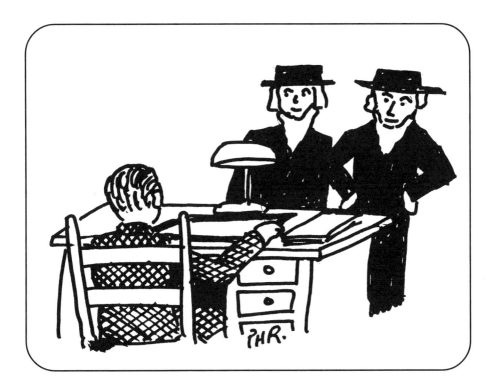

"NO PREMIUM" INSURANCE

In the 1950s and '60s, medical insurance and hospitalization insurance were increasing in their use among all people, except the members of the Amish faith. They really had the best insurance of all: helping each other—a type of community insurance, which satisfied their religion and tradition and which followed Jesus' teachings.

As I practiced medicine among the Amish, it was unusual for a church official to visit me and discuss the bill of a family unable to pay. The following story is about a rare encounter with this type of "no premium" insurance.

Eli and Rebecca Beiler, an Amish couple in their early forties, were active farmers. For some reason, they were unable to get ahead financially. They always had trouble paying their bills. Of their six children, I had delivered the last two, John and Sarah, three and five years earlier. Although I charged only $35 for each delivery in those days, and only $3 for an office visit, I had never received any payments for Rebecca's prenatal visits, the children's well-baby visits or Rebecca's deliveries. As with many Amish, well-baby visits were not made after the first one or two months.

The children had received no immunizations, although I had suggested them. At that time, diphtheria-pertussis-tetanus immunizations were the only immunizations available; for these we made only a $1 charge in addition to the $3 charge for the office visit. Polio vaccine had yet to be discovered; smallpox vaccination was required before entrance to school.

I saw the babies and children only when they were sick. With six children in the Beiler family, I was seeing at least one of them almost every month. When one child was ill, often several were, so there would be multiple visits for such ailments as measles, chicken pox, or severe upper respiratory illnesses. Their parents would not bring the children to the doctor for minor infections or injuries. When they came to my office, they had a bad injury or were seriously ill.

During the office visits, I frequently dispensed medicine which added to the charges the Beilers were incurring. Over a period of five to seven years, the family had accumulated a bill of $471 and had not made a single payment. The bills I sent them grew larger. In the past year, I had begun adding notes, requesting partial payment. Whenever I saw Rebecca with one of the children (I seldom saw Eli), I would ask about their ability to pay a little on the bill, or to pay for the present visit. Sometimes she would pay for the medicine in cash. But the bills continued to grow.

After the amount they owed me had gone unpaid for years, one evening Jacob Stoltzfus and Levi Fisher appeared in my office. Jacob said without preamble, "We came to see you about Eli Beiler's bill. We know it is high. We appreciate your caring for Eli and his family without payment up to this time. I have some of his medical bills here. I believe this is the last one, and it's for $471. Because we must pay the bill for him, we wonder how much you would be willing to accept as payment in full."

Although this was not to be the last time such a negotiation would take place with leaders of the Amish church, this was my first encounter with it. I was not sure what I should say. Nobody had prepared me for this type of bargaining. Finally, I said, "How would you feel about $350?"

Jacob asked, "Is that the best you can do?"

"That includes medicine which I had to pay for. I do not feel able to reduce the bill any further."

At that point, Jacob pulled out his checkbook, wrote a check and gave it to me. "Thank you, Henry. Thank you for taking care of the family. They are a fine family, but they never seem to be able to put any money back to take care of their medical expenses."

They went on their way. The Beilers had a clean slate.

This event is uncommon as Amish people are thrifty and industrious and are usually financially responsible.

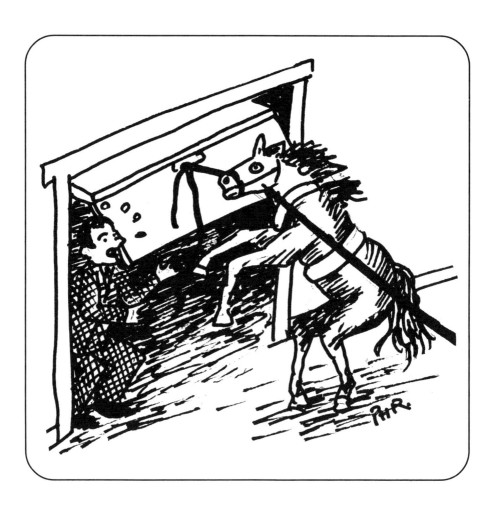

THE RISEN HORSE

In the midst of my busy office hours on a Thursday evening at 9:15, the phone rang. Isabel Harnish was requesting a house call for her sick husband, Andy. "Would you come out to see him tonight after you're finished in the office?"

She explained his symptoms and problems, and I said, "Yes. I should be there in one to one and a half hours."

I continued to see patients in the office. About 10 o'clock I started with the last of these, a little Amish girl, Sadie, who had been brought into the office by her mother, Rebecca. "What's wrong with Sadie?" I asked.

"She's had an earache that started last night and seems to be getting worse."

"Has she had fever?"

"I don't have a fever glass." That was Rebecca's term for a thermometer. "She seemed warm. She's had a cold all week."

I recorded the mother's answers, then began to examine Sadie. Seeing a red and bulging eardrum, I promptly confirmed an ear infection. I wrote the treatment measures on the record and said, "You're right. Sadie does have a severe infection in her ear. I'll give her an antibiotic. Continue it until it is gone. If she doesn't seem a lot better by Monday, let me know. Is she allergic to any medicine?"

Rebecca answered, "No."

After a few words of instruction, I said, "Good night" and was on my way to make a house call for Andy Harnish. I handed the records to my nurse, Nancy, as I picked up my bags and left the office. I knew that Nancy would give Rebecca the medicine I had prescribed and would provide directions about how to give it to Sadie, then would dismiss the two of them.

My office was in the lower floor of a split level house and our living quarters and garage were on the upper level. Hurrying to reach Mr. Harnish, I rushed up the steps, entered the garage and pressed the automatic door opener. I was greeted by the most awful, most wrenching shriek I had ever heard. Although it was dark outside, as the garage door went up I saw four hooves on the other side of the door. Rebecca's horse and carriage were tied to the garage door!

I pressed the door opener to reverse the door's direction and went outside to see if the animal was all right.

I re-entered the house and read the paper until Rebecca and Sadie departed. Then at last I left to see Andy Harnish.

And I never did mention to Rebecca the strange, uplifting experience her horse had undergone!

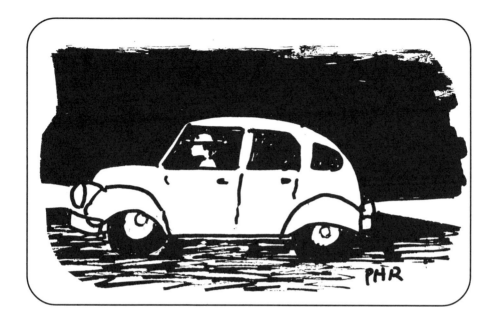

MY WIFE'S PROPHECY

The telephone rang about 1 o'clock one morning. I struggled from my sleep, sat up, rubbed my eyes, and answered the phone beside my bed. "Hello! Is this Dr. Wentz? My nephew is yelling and screaming and going crazy," a woman said. "Can you come and help him?" I could hear the noise over the telephone.

"I'll be right there. What's your address?" I dressed rapidly, opened the garage door, and drove to the east of town, half a mile away.

As I left the car I could hear the shouting, "Let me alone. I'll blast you to Kingdom Come."

A woman in a negligee and robe she had hurriedly thrown around herself opened the door for me. She appeared frightened. "I'm sorry I had to call you out at this hour, but we didn't know what to do."

I thought to myself, "What did I learn in medical school that can help in this situation? Nobody has ever turned me loose in a house with a madman. What do I do now?"

When we got upstairs, the woman said, "George, this is Dr. Wentz. He came to help you." I saw a young good-looking fellow, with every muscle well developed. He appeared taut, extremely tense, obviously up tight and upset. His uncle, the woman's husband, was holding him by the wrists to restrain him.

As I struggled to know how to respond to that introduction, I heard myself saying softly, "What's the matter? How can I help you?"

He shouted, "Get out of here! Who called for you? Who are you?" and kicked toward me as he continued to struggle against all of us and against himself.

I continued talking with him in a quiet voice but got back only incoherent replies, with obscenities and gestures of attack toward me.

Their pastor came in. He was a gentle graying man who had been pastor of their church for at least 35 years. He also attempted to quiet the young man, but with no more success than I had had.

It was about this time, around 2 a.m., that the phone rang, cutting through tension. It was my wife, Mary: "Rebecca's having her baby, and they need you right away."

Now I was forced to do something in a hurry to calm the young man. I got ready an injection of a barbiturate (this was before tranquilizers and anti-psychotic drugs were available). With the help of everybody there, I managed to bare the man's arm. I gave him the injection against his will, as he continued his violent attempt to escape. It was not the best approach. But nobody in my training had ever taught me how to take care of two emergencies at one time. This was the only solution I could come up with. I was only one person. I could not split myself in two.

Levi, Rebecca's husband, had been calling me almost daily for the last 10 days to tell me that his wife was ready to have her baby. She was having pain, he said, which was his way of announcing her labor had begun. From all indications, her time was near. Because of Amish religious practices Rebecca and Levi had no telephone, so I could never talk directly to her without taking a six-mile trip east of Strasburg to visit her home. I made this trip after each of her husband's calls, because she was being delivered at home; and each time I drove out there I determined that she was not in active labor. So when this latest telephone call came, my question was, "How urgent is this? Is she really in labor?"

My wife had awakened me during the previous night by saying, "Henry, I dreamed that Rebecca had her baby. You didn't get there in time. And when you did arrive, another physican from the other side of town was coming out of the house saying, 'Your baby is born. Everything is over. All is okay,' and you said, 'Thank you.'" At that point in the dream she awoke to give me this prophetic message. It certainly was not unusual for us to dream about Rebecca's big event, as so many of our daily activities had been interrupted by Levi's phone calls!

But now I was on one emergency and was being called to another; a woman in active labor at home is a definite emergency. I responded as rapidly as I could—first giving the young man an injection to sedate him, I hoped, and then dashing off to help this pregnant woman. I arrived at the site of the impending birth about 2:30 a.m. Right away I examined Rebecca.

"I've been having pains all night. I'm ready to have my baby," she said. My examination confirmed her statement. Her cervix was fully dilated, and the delivery should be imminent (she had given birth to four babies on previous occasions). Afterward, I could return to my other emergency. I sent Levi to boil water and get some of the necessities ready while I unpacked my instruments, gloves and other paraphernalia in preparation for the event. Remember, we were isolated with no telephone. Also, no electricity. We worked by the light of a kerosene lantern. There was no way I could communicate with my previous problem. This was in the days before radio pagers were available.

I waited. I waited. I waited and nothing happened. It seemed an hour. I know it was more than twenty minutes, and by now Rebecca had no pain. How could a woman have a baby without pain or contractions? Could a woman almost ready to deliver have no pain for this length of time?

Her abdominal wall was thin so I could easily palpate her uterus. She had poor abdominal musculature, and she had had four previous babies. I waited another five minutes, with my hand on her abdominal wall, but felt no uterine contractions. She had had no sedation or pain relievers.

I thought I remembered being taught in medical school that no woman had babies without increasing contractions of the uterus. My own experience gained through delivering more than 500 babies by this time, also made me think the results of my rectal examination were incorrect (we didn't do vaginal examinations at that time because of the possibility of introducing infection). Instead of the cervix being fully dilated, it may have been undilated and so thin it just felt fully dilated.

My mind kept vacillating. I was restless wondering about my very active young man with abnormal behavior. How was everybody getting along? And my job at the moment of helping a young woman have a baby—or was she ready? What should I do?

With my wife's prophetic dream on my mind, "You were late for the delivery," I left, saying to Rebecca, "I'll be back in half an hour. I need to check on another emergency in Strasburg."

By the time I returned to the original emergency, the young man had calmed down and the pastor had engaged him in conversation. He seemed somewhat coherent. I was just beginning to analyze the situation when the phone rang again. It was my wife: "Where have you been? I told you Rebecca needed you. Levi called again. It's urgent. Get there right away!"

While racing eastward at 3:45 a.m. on a deserted highway, with my eyes wide open I was praying, "Lord, help me to arrive in time. Alleviate her pain for ten minutes and I'll be ready."

I arrived. The local physician's car was there. As I got out of my car, he emerged from the house and greeted me, saying, "The baby is born. Everything is okay."

I replied somewhat sheepishly, "Thank you." I entered the house frustrated and embarrassed. What could I say?

To Rebecca I said, "I'm glad everything is all right. I'm sorry I left you. The doctor did a good job." The baby, wrapped in a blanket was crying lustily. Healthy lungs! I examined Rebecca and felt the firm postpartum uterus through her thin abdominal wall.

I examined the baby and found everything to be fine. I said, "I'll be back in a couple of days to see both of you."

Back home once more, I lay in my bed. I thought of the two simultaneous emergencies thrust upon me. I recalled my wife's on-target prophecy. I sighed, rolled over, and at last went back to sleep.

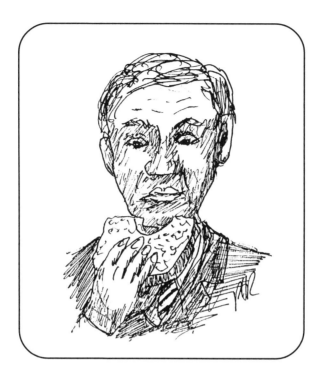

SURPRISE!

As I drove home for dinner my mouth was watering because of the gift Barbara had presented to me.

Naomi and Barbara Stoltzfus were two Amish maiden ladies who had lived together in Strasburg for a decade or more. Naomi, in her 60s, was known as "the cleaning woman." She enjoyed cleaning dirty, cluttered attics and basements. She not only did a good job of cleaning; she also frequently found places for things that were of no use to the families who had been hoarding them. Barbara, the older of the sisters, did the work around their house. Both worked hard and would toil on their family farm whenever help was needed.

As Barbara approached her mid-seventies, she developed heart failure. Since walking was the Stoltzfus sisters' principal means of transportation, and they could not readily come to my office, I would frequently visit Barbara at home. She took her medicine regularly. She also was on a low-salt diet. Naomi had taken over most of the domestic responsibilities by this time. She had baked a loaf of bread for me.

As I finished office hours that afternoon about 5, I anticipated the joy of eating this gift of bread. We ate dinner at 5:15 because I started working in the office again at 6 p.m.

After saying grace, I asked Mary for a slice of Naomi's delicious bread anticipating its delectability. I spread on butter and took my first bite. It tasted horrible. I looked surprised and asked my wife, "What's wrong with this bread?"

"I don't know. Let me taste it." She took one bite and exclaimed, "Do you have Barbara on a low-salt diet? The bread is made without salt. Now you know what a real low-salt diet tastes like."

Needless to say, I was tasting the fruit of my treatment and learning first-hand the poor flavor and flat taste of salt-free bread.

When I returned to visit Barbara and Naomi again, I thanked them for the delicious bread, which my family enjoyed in its entirety. I never wanted them to know about my confrontation with a piece of their low-salt diet. I expected them to continue eating the poor-tasting food for the sake of Barbara's health.

I discovered the flat taste and flavor of a salt-free diet. Little white lies helped my patients, I hoped, to comply with my instructions.

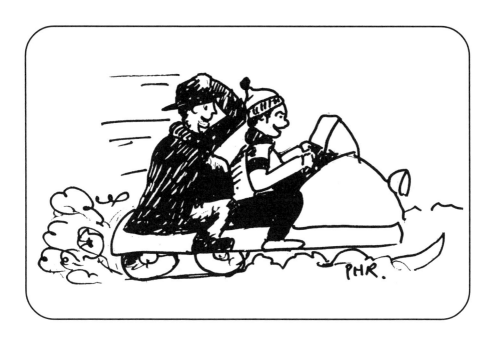

CURIOUS JONAS

Many Amish live on farms with long lanes that are unpaved dirt or mud paths. Because they don't use automobiles, they can become isolated, especially during snowstorms. During a particularly bad storm, with 12-14 inches on the ground and winds making roads impassable, I received a telephone call: "My neighbor, Jonas, has a chest pain. Can you come down?"

"How do I get there?"

"You can't get here in a car. Do you know where he lives?"

"Yes, I know. I'll get a snowmobile with a driver."

I called one of my neighbors, who had offered the use of his snowmobile for such circumstances. Without hesitation he asked, "When do you want to go?"

"Now."

"Okay, I'll be there."

I bundled up with a hat, scarf, heavy coat and galoshes and gathered everything I might need into two medical bags. We traveled over fields where roads were blown shut, with the wind and snow blowing in our faces. I wedged the two bags between the back of the driver and myself and held fast to his waist. Finally, we arrived at the isolated farmhouse.

I entered, took off my boots and some of my outer clothing, and went upstairs to see Jonas. He seemed more interested in the way I got there than in his own problem. He asked, "Henry, did you have any trouble getting here?"

"I came by snowmobile."

"You did. Do you have one?"

"No, a neighbor brought me. What's wrong with you?"

"I awakened early this morning with pain in my chest. I feel so tight. I have trouble breathing. Can you help me?"

I checked his blood pressure and pulse. His blood pressure, which usually had been 140/76 or so, was 90/60. His pulse was 92 beats a minute and regular. I examined his heart and lungs and heard a few crackles in the bases. His heart sounds seemed to indicate a potentially serious problem.

I said, "I believe you've had a heart attack, Jonas. You belong in the hospital."

His first comment was, "Oh no, I can stay at home." Then he thought about the pain he had encountered, "How are you going to get me there?"

"I must go home to use the telephone, but we can get the highway crew to open the road and get an ambulance out here. It really isn't safe for you to be here. It may be impossible for anybody to get to you tonight, if you stay here. You're pretty sick. Let me give you something for the pain and allow you to rest, and you stay in bed until the ambulance crew comes for you. Don't help them. Let them help you. They can carry you downstairs. I'll see you at the hospital. Remember: don't get out of bed! What cardiologist do you want?"

"You pick the doctor for me." I agreed to do so.

I walked downstairs, answered the family's questions, and returned home on the snowmobile. I telephoned the hospital to make arrangements, then called the local ambulance and highway crews to clear the snow from the highways and the farm lane so that Jonas could be taken to the hospital.

When I saw Jonas in the hospital later, he told me. "Henry, I disobeyed you. When you left the house, I just had to get out of bed to see you drive away on the snowmobile!"

Did Jonas' arising from his sickbed, against his doctor's orders, do him harm? Probably not, for he would live another ten years in generally good health. It's even possible that his zest for living, as exemplified by his curiosity about seeing me astride the snowmobile, could have helped him achieve his long, productive and happy life.

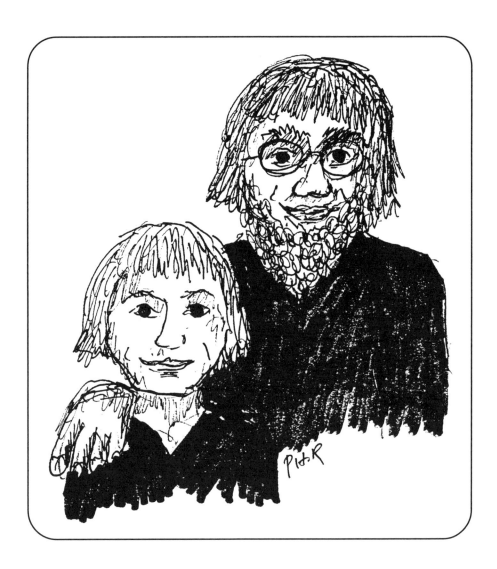

THE ARTIST ADDS
A FEW AMISH STORIES

by PAUL H. RIPPLE, M.D.

(Dr. Paul Ripple is my life-long friend. Over the years of my medical practice in nearby Strasburg I referred many patients, who needed eye care, to him. He is the illustrator of this book.)

One evening my wife and I were visiting a family about five miles south of the New Holland Pike, ten miles from Lancaster. We were forced to spend the night at the farm because of a severe snow-storm with drifting. The next morning I explained that I had patients in the Lancaster General Hospital that I had to see. My host bundled up and returned in an hour in an Amish sleigh. I then experienced a very colorful ride with an Amish friend over the hills, avoiding the roads that were drifted shut, to the New Holland Pike. From there I hitchhiked to the hospital.

———————

A handsome young Amish man named David had lost all of the central vision in each eye from a disease called toxoplasmosis. He had 20/200 vision in each eye, not nearly sufficient to pass a driver's test. I asked him, "How do you do your courting on Saturday nights?"

He answered, "My horse has good vision, much better than I do. He can make the decision to cross the street or highway."

―――――――――――

Most small children are afraid of doctors. In spite of all efforts, many scream, kick and become unmanageable. On some occasions I even need to arrange an examination under anesthesia. But this does not happen with Amish children. When mom or pop come into the room with the child, one remark from the parent and the child lies or sits perfectly still and fully cooperates with the doctor.

―――――――――――

An old Amish man from southern Lancaster County came to my office complaining that he was losing weight because he could not see well enough to shoot squirrels, which had become his main food. In the office I removed a pterygium, a growth that slowly grows over the cornea, from each of his eyes. A few weeks later I received a postal card from him explaining that he was now gaining weight.

―――――――――――

When the Amish are asked, "Do you have a phone number to make any change in appointments?" they usually give their non-Amish neighbor's phone number.

One Amish man said, "I have a phone in a little box on a telephone pole at the end of my lane. My dog hears the phone ring and comes to get me. Let the phone ring about twenty times."

One day an Amish father brought his seven-year-old son, Amos, to my office and said, "This boy can't read anymore. Last year he could read quite well. Since school started, he no longer seems able to read."

When I examined him, I noticed that he had very large pupils and that they did not constrict when I shone a light into them. Furthermore, he could not focus during near vision, a condition that is normal in people over fifty years of age (presbyopia), but very unusual in childhood (paralysis of accommodation).

Since this condition can follow a high fever, such as can be caused by scarlet fever, I asked, "Has Amos had any severe infection?"

When the father answered, "No," I noticed that he, too, had dilated pupils. When I called his dilated pupils to his attention, he replied, "My wife and I have needed our reading glasses much more frequently in the past few months."

I inquired, "What medications are you taking?"

The answer was, "None."

After much more questioning, the father volunteered, "Our family has been taking a health tonic, if you call that medicine. Each of us takes a tablespoon daily as we have every winter. We get this tonic from a salesman that comes to our door. In fact, this tonic is sold to a lot of Amish families to protect them from winter colds and other maladies."

"Would you tell me the name of this salesman, so I might call him and inquire about the contents of this tonic?"

I looked up his name in the telephone directory and called him. "What's in the tonic you sell door-to-door? Is there any atropine in it?"

He called back in a few minutes. "There is a little atropine in the tonic. Since you called, I went over my calculations and I misread a decimal point when I prepared the last batch, so it has ten times the amount it should have."

Atropine was first used several hundred years ago when ladies of the court put it in their eyes to dilate their pupils in order to make them look younger and more glamorous. It was first known as belladonna which means "beautiful woman."

The mystery of the inability to read and the dilated, fixed pupils had been solved.

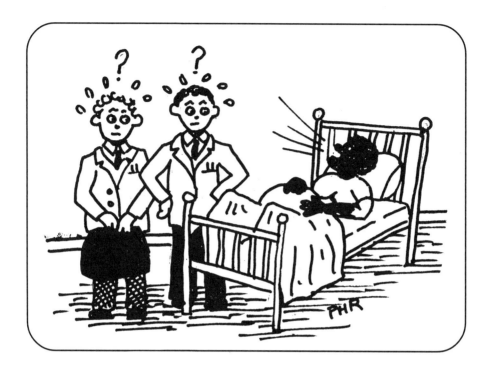

OUR FIRST TIME

At one point during our junior year in medical school, each student linked up with another. We went out to homes in central Philadelphia to assist women who were about to deliver babies. These women had been well screened and followed by obstetrical professors at the clinic. None of them was having her first baby, and none was having her 10th or more. None had any expected complications and none had trouble with previous pregnancies. So these pregnant women were as trouble-free as any could possibly be.

That was the theory, at least.

Each pair of students was given a bag that contained soap, washcloth, towel and razor. These articles were to enable us to prepare the patient for delivery. No syringe or injectable medication was available. In fact, the only medications in the bag were four aspirin tablets of five grains each and four ergotrate tablets of 1/65 grain each. (Ergotrate was used to contract the uterine musculature and inhibit bleeding after delivery.) Four pairs of sterile, patched and powdered gloves were available, as well as a bottle of finger cots for rectal examinations. We were not allowed to do any vaginal examinations in the home, because of the possibility of introducing infection. A lubricant was on hand, and two gowns, one for each of us, to protect our clothing. A bottle of sterile cord ties was in the bag with a pair of scissors and two hemostats; these were to be used to clamp the umbilical cord and to cut the cord and the cord tie after the delivery. Completing the collection was a small copper pan with a metal basket and top in which to place the instruments and sterilize them with boiling water while we waited for the woman to have her baby.

Fred and I were partners. We were called out of class one day and informed that Jenny, a potential mother assigned to us, was ready to have her baby. In those days we went by street-car to reach our destination. As we stepped off the trolley, we could hear screams, almost continuous, coming from the vicinity of the building for which we were looking. Fred looked at me. I looked at him.

"What's going on?" I asked.

"A woman's having a baby."

"We'd better hurry. It sounds as if she's having it right now!"

We rushed toward the source of the noise, and the number on the door corresponded to the number that was written on the paper that had been given us. We knocked and entered, not expecting anybody to respond to our knock. The sounds were really loud now. I remember thinking that everybody within a two-block radius of this place must be aware of the suffering. I wondered what they did at night. The whole neighborhood must be awakened when somebody was having a baby.

A man, the husband I assumed, saw us coming up the steps and motioned for us to hurry. We got to the top of the steps and couldn't even hear each other talk because of the screaming. I think we were both a little scared and anxious. We rushed into the room to which the man directed us. There, lying on a bed, sweating profusely —it was the middle of summer and the windows were opened wide —was a large woman. She was screaming at the top of her lungs. She interrupted her screaming long enough to say loudly, so the whole world could hear, "Doctors, you've got to help me. I can't stand this much longer. Hurry! Do something!" She resumed her screaming.

I was glad I was carrying the bag. This partially immobilized me. So it was up to Fred, who had both hands free, to run over and see what was happening. With all the screaming, both of us thought that the baby must be coming. He pulled up the sheet, expecting to see the vaginal opening completely obscured by the baby's head. But he saw no sign of an impending birth. Next, he placed his hands on her abdomen to feel the contractions of the uterus. But with her screaming, all he could feel were the tense abdominal muscles being used to express her misery.

By this time, I had placed the bag on the floor and opened it. I had sent the man, the identity of whom we had not established, to take the copper container with the instruments to the kitchen. I had instructed him to put water into the container and to place it on the stove, to boil the water and sterilize the instruments.

Now Fred called me over to a corner where we could talk. Believe me, this was difficult, with the patient yelling and Fred trying to keep his voice down so nobody else could hear. I finally heard him say, "I don't know what's going on. She's not having the baby, and I can't really tell much about her abdomen because of her screaming. You examine her. See what you think. You may want to examine her rectally, also, to try to determine what stage of labor she's in."

I said, "Thanks a lot!" Then I began trying to calm the woman enough to ask her a few questions and to examine her abdomen while her voluntary abdominal muscles were relaxed.

I said, "Now, Jenny, we're here to help you. Can you relax a little bit and answer some questions?" Without waiting for an answer, I asked, "How long have you been having so much pain? Is your pain continuous, or does it come and go, or get worse and then better?"

She responded, half yelling, "It seems like I've had this pain for hours and it's all the time. It doesn't let up. Can't you give me something for the pain? Doctor, Can't you help me?"

I was beginning to realize I wasn't going to get much help from her. Fred and I were going to have to figure this out ourselves. Maybe when the man returned from the kitchen he would be able to help us.

I again attempted to examine her abdomen. I spoke softly and calmly to her, to get her cooperation in the hope that she would stop screaming for a minute.

She did quiet down a little for a short time. As I tried to time any uterine contractions, her uterus did not feel hard and firm as I would have expected during labor; but every time she had a pain, she yelled and all her abdominal muscles contracted. I listened to the fetal heart as best I could, but it was hard to count because the mother's noise kept interfering with my hearing the faint sound of the baby's heart. Then I examined her rectally to try to determine how labor was progressing. This created even more piercing screams.

Once more I went over to the corner with Fred. I said, "You examine her and see what you think."

After his examination, which he performed along the same lines as I had done, he came over to me and said, "I don't think she's in labor."

I agreed with him. I said, "We have to do something about this horrible screaming. The people around here must think she's dying."

"What can we do?"

"We do have aspirin. Maybe that will help."

I went over to the patient and told her, "Everything seems fine. You are not going to have the baby right now. The baby seems okay. Its heart is beating fine. We are going to give you a pill now. If you still have pain in half an hour, you may have a second pill. If you still have pain an hour after the last pill, you may take the third pill. But don't take the third pill unless you absolutely need to, because this is strong medicine and we don't want you or your baby to have more of this medicine than necessary."

Then we walked over to the man and introduced ourselves. We discovered that, as we had thought all along, he was the woman's husband. We said to him, "We have given her a pill. Here are two more. If she still has pain in 30 minutes, give her a second one. If she still has pain an hour after you have given her the second one, you can give her the third pill. But don't give her the third one unless you absolutely need to, because we don't want her and her baby to have more of this strong medicine than absolutely necessary." We handed him a slip of paper. "Call us at this number in two hours and let us know how things are getting along."

We packed our bag and left the house. As we boarded the trolley to go home, we thought the noise had decreased considerably.

Two hours later her husband called and said, "Half an hour after you left, she was comfortable and fell asleep. She's been fine ever since."

About a week later, we were informed by another pair of medical students that this woman had delivered her baby. We had not been summoned because we were not on call for deliveries that day. The baby and mother were fine. They had experienced no complications. The mother had screamed loudly when she had labor pains and through the second stage of labor, but her team of medical students had handled things well.

That had been my first experience, and Fred's, with the strength of pain relief by aspirin—and the power of suggestion.

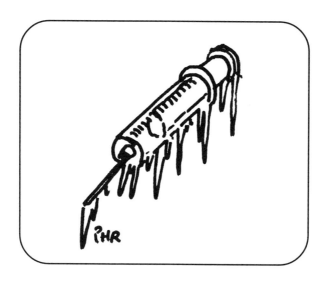

AN INTERN RIDES
THE AMBULANCE

Half a century ago interns rode in the ambulance with a nurse on every emergency call. I served as an intern in the mid-1940s, and I well remember making ambulance calls to train wrecks.

The first of these railroad accidents I had to deal with occurred about 3 a.m. on a bitter cold night. The crews had been shifting cars, coupling and uncoupling them as they delivered shipments to factories and warehouses. During this activity a gondola car ran into another freight car, stopping suddenly, shifting the load of steel plates in the gondola car against the opposite end. Just before the impact occurred, a railroad employee, the brakeman on the gondola car, had jumped down into it. When the steel plates shifted, they caught both of the brakeman's legs a few inches below the knees. They were almost completely crushed.

With a senior student nurse, Sally, and an ambulance driver, I reached the scene promptly. The temperature was hovering around zero, possibly lower. As I climbed into the railroad car, using the ladder attached to its side, I saw a man in extreme pain with both legs pinned between the end of the car and the steel plates. I asked Sally to hand me 1/4 grain of morphine sulfate in a syringe. She readied the morphine and climbed the ladder to give it to me. It took a few moments to find some bare skin through all of the man's clothing. Finally, I sank the needle into his bared lower arm a couple of inches above the wrist, but I was unable to push the plunger to inject the contents of the syringe. After several unsuccessful attempts, I removed the needle from his arm and returned it to the nurse. I asked her to give me another syringe with morphine sulfate. The same thing occurred. Then it dawned on me that the contents of the syringe were frozen. That was why I was unable to push the plunger to empty the syringe. Nobody had ever warned me about this in medical school or in my medical training. I wondered, "What do I do now?"

I said to the nurse, "Fill the syringe with 1/4 grain of morphine sulfate, then hold the loaded syringe against your body while you climb the ladder and until you hand it over to me. Give it to me immediately. Don't worry about sterility, if that's a problem."

We didn't have caps on the needles or disposable syringes. I'm not sure how many syringes we carried in our emergency bag. Anyway, Sally held the loaded syringe under her clothing against her warm body while she climbed the ladder. She removed the syringe from her torso and gave it to me, as I had requested. I was relieved to find that now I could push the plunger and unload the contents of the syringe. Finally, I was able to inject the pain reliever into the suffering victim.

While this was going on, I was busy talking to the train officials who had gathered. "How slowly can you pull these steel plates away from the end of the railroad car?"

"An inch at a time."

I could hardly believe this. The plates must have weighed several tons.

"Are you sure? We're talking about a man in here. We need to do this slowly."

They reassured me: "Let us do it. We can move this load an inch at a time."

Half an hour after we had given the pain killer to the victim, the train crew had their equipment in place. They said, "Tell us when."

In the meantime, Sally had handed me two rubber tourniquets. I had decided to wrap them around his legs below the knees over his clothing. It was so cold! I had thrown only an overcoat over my intern uniform, and I was shivering while I was trying to do all this.

I realized that I might not be able to cut off the man's circulation completely; but with the help of the cold temperature and the length of time his legs had been caught in this vise (it must have been more than an hour), blood loss might be minimal. Since he was still having so much pain, we injected another 1/4 grain of morphine before the move began. We had to use the same syringe, because we had no others; but I thought lessening pain was more important than sterile technique at this point.

When everything was ready, I informed the crew to go ahead. I was surprised that this rescue operation could proceed at such a slow pace and with such precision, as they separated the tons of steel from the end of the car. They moved the plates less than an inch at a time, while Sally and the ambulance driver (all of us were up in the railroad car by now) freed the man's dangling legs, tied them onto wooden splints, and placed him on a stretcher.

The railroad crew helped us lift the stretcher over the side of the car and carry the patient to the ground and then to the ambulance. Even in the warm ambulance, with all the clothing on this man, I was unable to check his blood pressure or even examine his legs at the place of injury. My thought was to get him to the hospital as soon as we could and to keep him as warm as possible; he must have been almost frozen during his exposure to the cold without being able to move. At the hospital I could turn him over to experienced physicians who could care for his specific needs under much more satisfactory conditions. Fortunately, we had been able to place the tourniquets below the knee.

He was forced to lose both legs below the knee, as I had expected, but the victim did survive.

I had learned that solutions, even morphine, can freeze. But I also had found that the warmth of a human body can be used to conquer this problem.

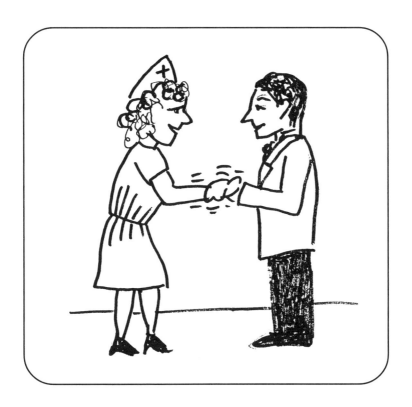

A TRAIN WRECK
IN PARADISE

My first ambulance ride to a train wreck had been the aftermath of a freight train mishap; the second time was for a passenger train accident.

I was on a rotation for the receiving ward (that's what we called the emergency room at that time). We had just repaired a large laceration of a patient's lower leg. During this procedure, I had become upset with the staff nurse, Minnie, because she had taken so long to get the instruments I needed. I was afraid the effects of the novocaine would wear off before the operation was completed. As a result, I had yelled at the nurse and had shown hostility toward her. She was upset. I was infuriated.

When you're an intern, the most important person in your medical life is the nurse—even more important sometimes than the attending physician. After all, the nurse has experience; for years she has been dealing with patients who have problems and has been working with the staff physicians. She knows the best way to handle a particular predicament and also knows the way in which each attending physician prefers to evaluate and treat certain problems.

I had completed my medical education at Jefferson Medical College about two months previously; and I was unfamiliar with many of the medical and surgical problems I saw, except to the extent I had encountered them in medical textbooks.

It was at this time that an emergency call came in about a passenger train wreck at Leaman Place, near Paradise. Several passengers had been injured. How many, or how badly, no one yet knew. The ambulance driver, a helper and the staff nurse, Minnie, would be accompanying me on this trip. I was going off into the unknown with a nurse who was fuming at me, and she would know more than I about how to handle an emergency with multiple people injured. I needed all the help I could get.

Another multiple-injury accident had occurred within the past year. At that time the receiving ward personnel had recommended that a label be attached to each patient; on this tag would be recorded his or her injuries, any medications used and the dosage and time they were administered. Those were the days of no two-way communication. If for some reason the intern did not return to the hospital with the victims, the personnel in the receiving ward might have no knowledge of the type of injury or the medication that had been given. The tags provided that vital information.

As we approached Paradise, I tried to carry on a conversation with Minnie. I speculated about what we would find at the accident scene and how we might prepare to handle the emergency. When I asked her for suggestions, she responded, "Well, Dr. Wentz, you seem to know everything. I don't see why you need my help for this. I just came along for the ride." Things were not off to a promising start!

We were now within a few minutes of the wreck and she was still reacting like this. What should I do? I tried to reason with her on the basis of her wealth of experience: "Look, Minnie, you have had much more practice than I with accidents of this magnitude. I'm sorry. Let's work together for the sake of the people who are injured. You demonstrate your Florence Nightengale Pledge, and I'll try to live up to my Hippocratic Oath."

Before she could reply, we were there. I still wasn't sure whether her feelings had changed, but I hoped. By this time we could see the wrecked trains, two of them, and people at the scene directed us to the worst areas. All of us got out of the ambulance, and each was sent to a different area for different victims. With emergency bag in hand, I ran to the victim who was supposed to be in the worst shape. Minnie took a few supplies and went in another direction. The driver and helper went with others to assess the extent of injuries to the victims. They were to report back to us with their evaluation. The victim I was to treat had been trapped by the wreck in the men's room of a passenger car. I found him wedged between the walls of the small room, with one foot caught. In addition, one of his arms was injured.

After inquiring about his reaction to medications and any allergies, I injected morphine into his uninjured arm. I briefly examined him further, then splinted and bandaged his injured leg and arm. The railroad crew now was able to move the damaged car slowly to release his foot.

I recorded on the tag attached to the victim the medication and dosage he had received and the time it was given, and I noted the injuries to his leg and arm.

By this time Minnie had arrived to help me with the other victims and to tell me about the woman they had taken her to see. Another ambulance had arrived (in those days hospitals provided the only ambulances, and there were no trauma centers). We had two stretchers in each ambulance. By allowing the least injured to sit in seats—one with the driver and one in the back—we were able to transport four patients in one ambulance and three in the other. We saw only seven people injured sufficiently to warrant the use of ambulance transportation. Because the second ambulance carrying Minnie and me did not return to the hospital for at least half an hour after the first ambulance had arrived at the receiving ward, the patients' tags containing medical information proved invaluable.

The scene of the accident and the number of injured victims had evidently melted the negative feelings the nurse and I had had for one another. While we worked together as a team with the driver and helper, neither Minnie nor I spoke any harsh words. I'm not sure my last mitigating words to her had helped, but I believe we both felt overwhelmed by the task before us.

In addition to the seven victims we sent in the ambulances, we saw 10 or 12 others with minor bruises or injuries. To these we gave first aid. We examined their injuries, cleansed them with soap and water, and applied merthiolate and bandages. You must remember that this was in the days before the threat of malpractice suits caused any problems, and we felt comfortable taking care of the victims at the scene without any follow-up or further studies. In addition, by the time we finished our work, the authorities had buses ready to transport the rail passengers to their destination, Philadelphia or Harrisburg, and the people we helped were able to continue their journey without further interruption.

This accident was a great educational experience. We were directed to the more seriously injured first. The entire medical team worked together. I learned the value of controlling my feelings when I was frustrated. I had already been aware of the importance of a nurse and other experienced medical personnel, but this experience provided me with a reminder that their friendship and cooperation were as valuable as their experience.

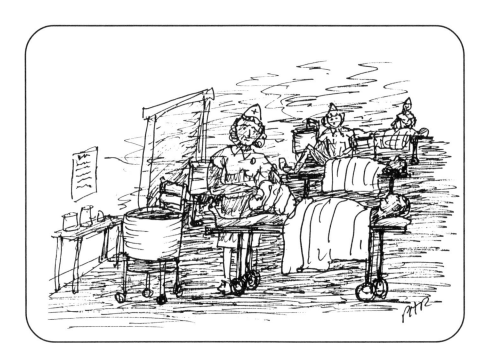

POLIOMYELITIS

IN THE 1950S

Shortly after I started my medical practice in 1948 at Strasburg, Pennsylvania, I was asked to assist in the care of patients who were victims of poliomyelitis at the Lancaster General Hospital. I was a member of a staff of three physicians; Dr. Edgar Meiser was the chief, Dr. Louise Slack was the pediatrician and I, as a family physician, was assistant to both.

Poliomyelitis (infantile paralysis) was one of the most dreaded diseases of childhood during this era. Each year brought fear to families with children. Prior to 1960 swimming pools, theaters and other public places where families gathered were sometimes closed to aid in the prevention of the spread of this plague.

A polio unit was established in a portion of the hospital with private and semi-private rooms and four-bed wards. The Pennsylvania Department of Health designated this as the unit for Lancaster County, and later Lebanon County was included. Each summer we were busy caring for young adults, babies and children with symptoms of polio. From August through October, it seemed that everybody who had upper respiratory or gastrointestinal symptoms with a stiff neck was admitted to our unit for observation and diagnosis. As a result, it was a great learning and teaching experience. We saw a variety of illnesses: tetanus, meningitis, infectious mononucleosis, tularemia, multiple sclerosis, sore throats, ear infections, mastoiditis, encephalitis, rheumatic fever, pneumonia and many more.

New patients were kept in private rooms until a definite diagnosis was made or poliomyelitis was definitely excluded. A confirmative diagnosis of polio was made on the basis of the symptoms, stiff neck, occasional weakness of a muscle group, and examination of spinal fluid. Polio patients were admitted to the polio unit. If polio was excluded, the patients were either discharged or transferred to the appropriate area of the hospital.

With financial help from the March of Dimes, instituted by President Franklin D. Roosevelt, and other agencies, the Lancaster General Hospital purchased an iron lung. Others were added later. At one time the hospital had five of these in operation.

I distinctly remember the helplessness all of us physicians felt as we watched the disease progress in some patients to weakness or paralysis of a limb or limbs to involvement of the nerves controlling the respiratory function to the bulbar (critical) area of the brain. Patients who experienced this rapid progression of symptoms frequently continued to death while the medical personnel stood by with no knowledge of what to do to avoid the end result.

Dr. Meiser became an expert in determining the need for assistance in breathing, and the only assistance we had was the bulky, large respirator, known as the iron lung. At this time studies of pulmonary function and blood gases were unknown, so clinical judgment was our only guide. Many patients fought this method of assisted breathing, which only made their condition worse. Dr. Meiser frequently gave sedatives to overcome the patient's severe anxiety and to get his or her cooperation. Once a patient was placed in the iron lung, he or she either progressed to bulbar involvement and death or remained in this respirator for months, if not indefinitely. After the acute phase subsided and the patient's condition had stabilized, attempts were made to gradually wean the patient from this massive instrument. The process took weeks. It required a lot of patience and the cooperation of the patient with concerned doctors and nurses. Although the patient's head remained outside of the iron lung, the remainder of the body was enclosed. Two portholes on each side were the only entries to give nursing care, and these openings with rubber closures were limited in size so that the attendant's arms would close the gap and not allow air pressure to escape from the machine. A larger opening on one side was available for use; but it could be opened only for a few seconds, or the negative and positive pressure produced by the machine would be lost and then the patient would receive no assistance in breathing.

As soon as the diagnosis was established, the patient's back, neck and extremities were placed in "hot packs." These comprised flannel material soaked in heated tubs. The hot cloths were wrapped onto the patients' limbs and kept in place with pins. The purpose of the hot packs was to relieve the patients' spasms and pain. This treatment had been started by Sister Kenny; and Edna Schreiber, a registered nurse and therapist, had been sent to Minnesota to learn the technique. In addition, Miss Schreiber had learned from Sister Kenny exercises for muscle re-education. This therapy was given to each patient who had any weakness or paralysis to help him or her regain function of the affected muscles.

In 1954 the census of the poliomyelitis unit in the hospital had reached its peak. There were 118 patients admitted with possible poliomyelitis and 80 patients finally diagnosed as definitely having polio. Of these, 28 were paralytic, 38 non-paralytic and 14 had bulbar involvement. In later years it was discovered that many of these non-paralytic patients did not have poliomyelitis, but were infected with Coxsackie or ECHO viruses. Of the 80 patients, 62 were able to return home, four died and 14 were transferred to other units or other hospitals.

In 1958 no polio patients were admitted until late in the year, when two came in. Gamma globulin was found effective to prevent paralytic polio in 1952, and thousands of children were given this injection. In 1955 the killed vaccine discovered by Dr. Jonas Salk was administered to children. In 1962 Dr. Meiser directed the local program of immunization of thousands of children and adults at the local schools by the live orally administered polio vaccine developed by Dr. Albert B. Sabin. The polio unit at the Lancaster General Hospital was phased out, to everybody's delight and relief; this dreaded disease had been conquered.

During the years when the threat of polio was raging, we had dealt with numerous memorable cases. Here are four of them.

Johnny was about six months old when his mother, Anne, noticed he was eating poorly; he had vomited a couple of times and seemed irritable. Anne, a nurse, found Johnny's temperature to be moderately elevated. Within 48 hours she thought she noticed a lack of movement in his left arm. She brought him to see me. I confirmed her findings and noticed some stiffness of his neck, decreased reflexes in his extremities, and some apparent weakness in his left arm or unwillingness to move it. He was admitted to the polio unit, where the diagnosis was confirmed by examination and laboratory studies that included the spinal fluid examination.

Johnny was placed in hot packs and later encouraged to use his left arm, hand and fingers. Muscle re-education in a six-month-old infant was not practical, but exercises and encouragement to use his left arm eventually resulted in an almost complete return of its function.

Marie, a young married woman with children, had a mild upper respiratory infection with headache and fever. She was examined by a physician and found to have a stiff neck and decreased patellar reflexes bilaterally and some weakness of her left leg. When she was admitted to the polio unit, the diagnosis of polio was confirmed.

It was frustrating to all of us physicians and other medical personnel to watch the rapid advancement of more serious symptoms as she lost the ability to use her arms and legs, then began to have difficulty in breathing. Based on our clinical evaluation, we determined her need for respiratory help. She had to be placed in an iron lung. In the beginning she fought the large machine and was unable to adjust her limited breathing ability to the positive and negative pressure of the apparatus. Sedation made it easier for her until she became accustomed to the rhythm of the instrument, and then her respiratory movements could synchronize with it.

Marie received excellent nursing care. Nurses changed her position and exercised her paralyzed limbs. They placed her in hot packs, bathed her, and cared for her vital functions through the port-holes on each side of the iron lung.

Really she was almost totally helpless, although she was able to talk and communicate with us. After months of treatment, we could see virtually no progress. She had to be fed; her four limbs were paralyzed; she was unable to breathe without assistance. She was moved to a respiratory assistance center at Baltimore. This move was quite an event. A large truck transported Marie's iron lung. State police provided an escort. Pennsylvania Power and Light Company provided the electrical energy to operate the medical equipment during her journey. Nurses accompanied her to care for her needs. She lived the rest of her life with respiratory assistance. But she lived.

Ruth, an active adolescent, was admitted with the disease. She received the usual treatment—bed rest, hot packs, and later muscle re-education. She was a happy girl, always smiling.

She had noticed a little weakness in her left leg. In fact, one of the first happenings that aided the diagnosis was a fall on the way to the bathroom. Quite a few young people had experienced this. Dr. Meiser would remind us, "If a patient falls on the way to the bathroom, he or she probably has polio." With continued therapy and learning to use her muscles to extend her foot and her toes, Ruth regained a great deal of her muscle strength. She was discharged and fitted with a special shoe and brace to correct her foot drop. She was able to walk again.

Elmer, an active businessman, was admitted in an acute stage of his disease with weakness in all of his limbs. He rapidly developed paralysis of his respiratory muscles and diaphragm and was placed in the iron lung. In spite of all of this help, the disease progressed to his brain, with bulbar involvement. He died within a week of the onset of his disease, while we stood helplessly by.

––––––––––––––––

These patients are a cross-section of the people we saw with infantile paralysis or polio.

Prevention by polio vaccine came too late for them. But as the end of the 20th Century nears, polio is rapidly following smallpox as an extinct disease on our globe.

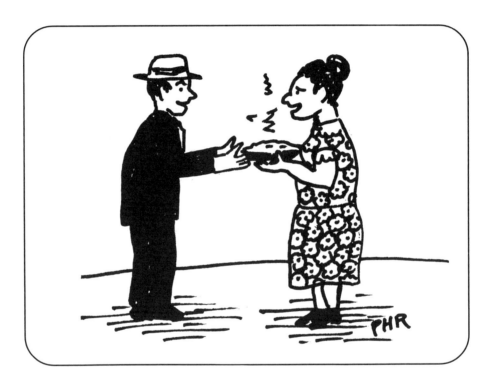

HEART FAILURE

"Sally is filled up again and needs to have fluid removed. When can you come down to do it?" Esther, Sally's mother, said over the telephone.

"I'll plan to do it at 11 tomorrow morning, and I'll try to stop between 10 and 10:30 to give her an injection," I replied.

To ease her anxiety and discomfort, I usually gave Sally an injection of morphine thirty minutes to an hour before I performed an abdominal paracentesis (removal of fluid from the abdomen) at her home. As I hung up the telephone, I thought with empathy of Sally and her serious problems. And I thought of my own frustration at having to carry out this procedure every three to four weeks without her ever getting better.

Sally, 27 years old, had had several bouts of rheumatic fever in her childhood and adolescence. Rheumatic fever affects many parts of the body, but most especially the heart. The illness follows a bout of streptococcal infection, usually a sore throat. Some strains may affect the kidneys; but much more common, in the days before antibiotics and sulfonamides, was the effect on the heart muscle and more seriously, the valves. Sally had heart failure as the result of damage to the valves of her heart from recurring attacks of this disease.

En route to another house call the next morning, I stopped to give Sally her injection and said, "In about 45 minutes I'll return with my wife to tap your abdomen."

After completing my other visit I returned to get my wife, Mary, who although not a nurse had learned to assist me in many ways.

It was a beautiful spring day as we drove from our home-office combination in Strasburg toward our destination. The leaves were budding and the birds were singing. But I couldn't get my thoughts off a pretty girl, made an invalid by disease, who really had no opportunity to enjoy the out-of-doors except through the window and through repetition of the same scenes through the changing seasons. My wife and I discussed the life this young girl faced and her reactions to us. She always greeted us with a smile, although I'm sure she dreaded each operation.

I told Mary, "I remember the first time I ever saw this procedure done. It was in Jefferson Hospital in Philadelphia. An intern, a couple of resident physicians and a few medical students like me were watching a skilled physician perform this surgery under sterile conditions, with an experienced nurse in attendance to assist the doctor. As he made the incision he told us of all the potential dangers. 'I could perforate the bowel or bladder. Always have the patient empty his or her bladder before the procedure. I could injure the liver or blood vessel or other vital parts. Infection could develop.' He made it look so easy as he inserted the instrument, and out flowed the fluid."

The first time I did this at home on Sally I thought of all these possible problems and how alone I was with no trained medical personnel to help if anything went wrong. Now I had done this many times and felt more confident, and I am sure the patient and family also felt confidence in me, with so many successful punctures behind us.

These were the "good old days?" of medicine, when the only diuretics were mercurials given by injection to enhance the functioning of the kidneys so they would put out more urine. The injections were preceded by four days of large horse-pill-size doses of ammonium chloride (two pills four times a day) to acidify the urine and to increase the efficiency of each injection. Such medications were not nearly as powerful as today's oral diuretics, and a sore spot was produced at the site of the injection as a result of the local irritation from the drug. Digitalis, mercurials and sedatives were our main armamentarium against heart failure. A special diet, low in salt, and physical and mental rest were other aids in combating the problem. When these failed we had to use surgical procedures to assist in the removal of excess fluid.

The little village about three miles from the center of Strasburg consisted of a village store, a one-room school and a few houses, in addition to a couple of house trailers. Sally lived in a two-story frame house on a seven-acre farm, with a small barn along the road. We parked our car in front of the barn and carried our bags up the narrow concrete walk to the house.

I said, "Hello, everybody!" as my wife and I entered through the kitchen. This room was the main room in the house. It was where people congregated when they weren't watching television in the adjoining parlor. Esther was always there. She was a great help to us. She took excellent care of her married daughter and provided her with a lot of much-needed support. Sally's two sisters also were there, but they usually made themselves scarce when this surgical procedure was going on. They were 10 and 15 years respectively. Sally's husband, Bob, would help when he was at home and not working at an industrial plant in Lancaster. They had married a few years previously in spite of Sally's health, during a time when she was feeling better and thought things might work out differently for them. Bob was attentive to her and seemed to be loving and compassionate through her prolonged illness. Sally's father was frequently working at a feed mill in Lancaster; but today he was busy on their small farm and truck patch, where he grew tobacco and also some of the food they ate.

To help entertain the patient and the rest of her family which of course was rendered relatively immobile because of Sally's condition, the family had recently bought a parakeet. Unknown to me, the bird was out of his cage and was flying around the room when I entered. I spotted it at once. With my voice tinged with anxiety, I asked, "Won't you please put that bird in its cage? I can't stand a bird flying around my head."

This apprehension must be a carryover from my childhood. I remember that my grandfather would catch a chicken in the chicken house in our backyard. Then he would put its neck over a wooden stump placed there for that specific purpose and chop off its head with a hatchet. The head would fall off the stump while the rest of the chicken flitted around on the ground in a meaningless way, blood flying every which way. That image dominated my mind every time a bird flew close to me, especially in a limited enclosure.

Sally was incapable of walking up and down steps, so her bedroom was downstairs adjoining the parlor. As my wife and I entered Sally's room, we were greeted by the usual smile and a pleasant "Hello." She was sitting as erect as possible in her bed.

I replied, "Hello, how are you doing? We came to remove the fluid in your belly that is causing you so much discomfort."

"Thank goodness! I can't stand this another day."

Sally's mother and Mary got things ready while I did a last-minute examination of the patient. Her face was lean and drawn. The veins in her neck were distended. Her heart was greatly enlarged and, although the rhythm was regular, I heard murmurs all over her chest. Fortunately, her lungs had stayed relatively clear; but I easily palpated her enormous, engorged liver. I saw and felt it pulsating as a result of a valvular dysfunction (tricuspid insufficiency) from her disease. I saw and felt marked ascites (fluid in her abdomen), as well as edema of her back over her sacrum. As usual, she had emptied her bladder before I had arrived, so her bladder was not palpable. The scars on her abdomen were chronic and multiple as a result of many procedures.

We undertook paracentesis only when Sally felt too uncomfortable from the accumulation of fluid and requested that it be done. There was some swelling of her lower legs and ankles, although she maintained that at a minimum by keeping her feet elevated for long periods at a time.

Her mother brought in a basin from the kitchen. Closed drainage procedures were uncommon or unheard of at this time. Today fluid is removed from a body cavity into a sealed container. Mary helped Sally to sit up, with her legs hanging down from the bed and her feet firmly planted on the floor. On the opposite side of the bed we turned a wooden kitchen chair upside down and placed it against her back, with a pillow between her back and the chair, to support her during the procedure. At the foot of the bed I placed the sterile drape with the instruments, now unwrapped, laying on it.

Next I cleansed Sally's abdominal wall and applied merthiolate. After washing my hands at the sink with soap and water, I put on sterile gloves and placed a sterile drape with an opening in the center over her lower abdomen. Her mother took her position at Sally's back, supporting her by holding the chair and pillow against her. "Are you comfortable, Sally?" she asked. "Is there anything I can do to make it easier?"

"Are you ready, Mary?" I inquired as I filled the syringe with novocaine.

"Yes," said my wife, "I have the basin here."

I made an injection into the scarred area of the abdomen, and the surgery had begun. A short time later I made a one-inch longitudinal incision and inserted a trochar (a sharp pointed instrument run through a metal tube with a spout on the end). As soon as I removed the insert, fluid began to flow under gravity from Sally's peritoneal cavity into the basin held below.

"Are you comfortable? Am I hurting you?" I asked.

"Are you feeling okay? Can I push you up a little more?" her mother asked.

"I'm tired, but I feel all right. Oh, that hurts!" said Sally. I had changed the position of the trochar a little to improve the flow of the fluid and probably had pierced an adhesion.

"I'm sorry. I think everything will be all right now."

When the basin became full, I plugged the flow until it had been emptied and returned. The results, usually measuring one to two quarts, would be discarded. After I drained the fluid, I removed the trochar, inserted a stitch to close the incision and put a bandage in place. Sally resumed her former position. I examined her heart, vital signs, lungs and abdomen again to make certain everything was in satisfactory condition.

We knew nothing at that time about measuring electrolytes. Certainly, electrolytes in her body were altered by the diuretics and the removal of fluid. Fortunately, from the electrolyte standpoint, the diuretics in our armamentarium at the time were not sufficiently strong to change significantly their concentration in body fluids, compared with the powerful oral diuretics used today.

In the early '50s the total cost for this procedure was $15. That included the morphine injection, novocaine for anesthesia, sterile surgical instruments, Mary's help and the surgery itself as well as the preoperative and postoperative evaluation. We needed no code number, and we had to fill out no forms. No "third party," such as a government agency or insurance company invaded the intimacy of the physician-patient relationship. Only the patient's family and the physician were involved in the economic part of medicine. Likewise, only the patient, the patient's family and the physician participated in the clinical aspects. Later, insurance did pay for this procedure.

By the time we were finished, willing hands had prepared the noon meal and the sisters had the table arranged in the kitchen. Betty, the youngest sister, said, "I'm glad it's over. I hate that."

Richard, the father, came in from the field ready to eat. "Hi! How did everything go?" he greeted us. "How are you feeling, Sally?"

Sally replied, "Okay. It's over." She would now rest for a while and eat a special meal a little later.

As we left, Esther gave us a cherry pie (my favorite kind). "Enjoy this. I baked it this morning."

"Thank you," I said, "This is the best part of the whole thing." She knew how to make good cherry pie, and I was already looking forward to the next one.

As Mary and I re-entered the bright spring sunshine, we were aware once more of our good health and the beauty of the day. We also were happy that things had gone well and that we were able to provide some relief, at least for a few more weeks, for Sally.

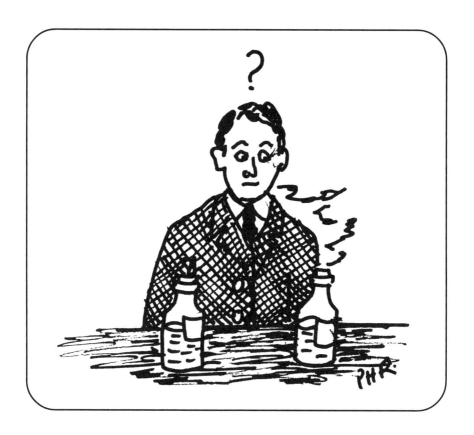

THE WRONG MEDICINE

The Stovers were a prominent family of business people in the small town of Strasburg. One family member was well known in the community but had an unfortunate problem with alcohol, a problem that was kept as secret as possible in the 1950s.

Shortly after I started general practice in Strasburg, Richard Stover's wife, Jane, telephoned and asked me to visit her husband. On winding roads I traveled one or two miles from the village into the countryside. At the Stover's property a paved driveway led to a beautiful colonial house that could not be seen from the road. This house was set on a farm with rolling hills, fertile fields and woodlands which deer, squirrels, rabbits and many birds called home and their place of play. Richard was a gentleman farmer who had somebody else till the soil and grow the grain and tobacco and corn.

As I entered the house, Richard said, "Hello Doc-doctor, h-how are you?"

"I'm fine," I answered. "What can I do for you?"

"I-I d-don't need anything. Who-who c-called for you?"

"Your wife called. Thought maybe I could give you something to help settle you down."

As he was pacing the floor, unable to sit still, he replied, "I'm c-calm. L-look at my arms. See-see h-how st-still they are." In fact, his arms and hand were full of tremor. But he plunged ahead, blustering, "I-I d-don't n-need anything from y-you."

"What did you have to drink this morning?"

"I-I j-just had a lille n-nip this-this m-morning. I-I'm fine. Y-you go see-see s-some s-s-sick p-patients."

"I came to help you. Let me give you a sedative and then you can go and rest a little."

"I-I d-don't n-need any er-rest. I-I sl-slept all night."

As we talked, more and more it became apparent that the best immediate treatment would be a sedative to calm him down. In those days the best medication for sedation of alcoholics was paraldehyde. Since I did not have any with me, I said, "I'll go and see "Doc" Schott and get something for Jane to give you." I intended to return to Strasburg and obtain some from the drugstore, which was located next door to my home-office combination.

"No! You g-go t-tend t-to your oth-other p-patients. I-I'll b-be all right."

Jane had come into the room. "Now, Dick, let the doctor help you. You know you need some help. He's just going to give you a sedative and let you sleep a little. You'll feel better afterwards."

"I'm fi-fine. Why did you call him and waste his t-time?"

Jane followed me to the door. I asked her, "Can't you keep liquor away from him?"

"I try really hard. But he gets on the phone and calls a friend and they smuggle it in to him when I'm not looking or when I'm away."

"I'll get the medicine and I'll be back in a few minutes," I said.

I got into the car and drove a couple of miles into Strasburg. Since the pharmacist was a neighbor, I had gotten to know him. "Doc" Schott, as he was called, was a little old man with a tradition in Strasburg. He went with the town. Had been born and raised there. Knew everybody—and everything about them.

Tall shelves stood along each wall, with some medications in the old-fashioned labeled jars. I also saw many more containers with all kinds of vegetable and flower seeds. Boxes of candy, many bottles and cans of patent medicines, and other things you can find in pharmacies including toothpaste, deodorants and greeting cards. To the rear was a large oak panel that separated his working area from the remainder of the store, and he was the only person who knew what went on back there.

When I entered nobody else was in the store. When "Doc" peered around the large panel in the rear, I inquired, "Do you have any paraldehyde you could give me?"

"How much do you want?"

"Give me four ounces."

He went back into his work area where I could no longer see him or what he was doing and returned in a few minutes with a package wrapped in white paper containing what appeared to be a four ounce bottle. "Thanks," I said. "Charge it to me."

I returned to the Stover residence immediately, thinking not only about the delay to them but also about all the things I had to do that morning before lunch and the beginning of office hours at 1 p.m.

As I entered triumphantly with my package, I greeted Jane, "I got the medicine. Here it is." As I started to open the package, I gave instructions to Jane: "Give him two teaspoonfuls now, and one teaspoonful every two to three hours until he is calmed down. After he rests a while he should be all right. Get rid of all the alcohol in the house."

By this time I had opened the package and given it to her. Just before I turned to leave, I had a suspicious thought. I said, "Give me that." I opened the bottle to smell it. Paraldehyde has such a distinctive odor that if you've smelled it once you'll never forget it. In fact that was its great disadvantage: it was excreted through the lungs, and the odor was overwhelming. You could tell anybody who had had it in the past few hours. As soon as I sniffed the bottle, I knew that "Doc" Schott had not given me paraldehyde but formaldehyde, an entirely different drug used in the past for embalming.

Immediately I took the medicine from Jane, wrapped it up again, and excused myself. "I need to take this back to 'Doc.'" I ran out the door and drove back to town.

Again at the pharmacy I said, "I asked for paraldehyde. You gave me formaldehyde. Do you have paraldehyde?"

"Yeah." He took the bottle from me and in a few minutes was back with another bottle.

When he started to wrap it, I said, "Don't bother. Let me smell it and I'll take it this way."

Again I was on my way back to the farm in the country, this time with the correct medicine.

"Here's the medicine," I yelled to Jane. I wrote the directions on the label as I instructed her again. "Good-bye, Richard. Listen to Jane. Take your medicine and stay away from liquor."

"You seem to be under the false impression that I-I d-drink a l-lot. I only have an occ-occasional d-drink. I-I d-don't d-drink much. You-you go-go see-see y-your sick p-patients."

I handed her the medicine and left, wondering whatever made me smell that medicine in the first place. As I drove to see my next patient at home, I thought to myself, "You know, if I hadn't smelled that medicine, I'd be leaving town in a hurry, and I've been here only a little over a year!"

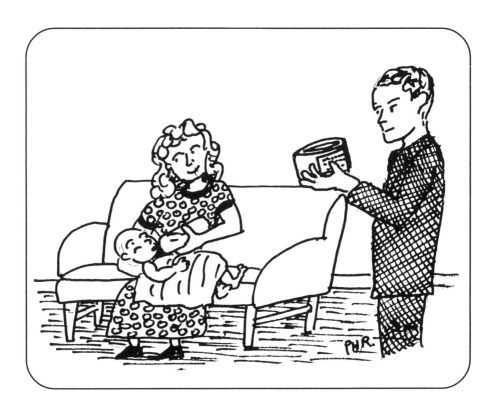

A LOST OPPORTUNITY

In my practice, newborn babies were not a rarity.

John was the product of a normal delivery to a proud and happy mother and father. He left the hospital at one week of age as a healthy newborn. I had given the usual instructions to his mother for the care of her first-born child.

The routine one-month well-baby checkup showed no abnormality. Mother, father and John were doing fine. John's mother believed that her milk supply was dwindling, and both parents wished to have the child on formula. So this I instituted according to their desire when my pleas for continuing nursing seemed to fall on deaf ears. They had been talking about this for days, even weeks, and in their minds the decision had already been made to discontinue nursing John.

One night the unrelenting sound of the emergency office bell awakened me. I was surprised to see these parents, with their child in convulsions.

Few things are more devastating to parents and physician alike than a convulsing child. I remember being told in medical school that if one is called to see a child with convulsions, "Tell the mother to cool the child with cold water. Hopefully, the convulsions will have ceased by the time you arrive. Then you can examine the child and calmly advise the family what should be done." But here the child had been brought to the office in a seizure. And John did not seem hot, as would have been the case in a convulsion brought on by fever. In fact, after he was settled down and the convulsion ceased, everything seemed fine. His temperature was normal, and the complete examination was normal for a two-month-old infant. What could the problem be? John had no history of a fall or injury nor any antecedent symptoms that would account for his convulsions. I reassured the parents and told them of things to watch for, and sent the family home.

I was alarmed when a couple of weeks later, in the middle of the night, they again appeared at my office door with John in the same situation. Acting quickly, I gave him anticonvulsant medication. Then I examined him, with the same results as before. Apparently the child's condition was normal. This time, though, I admitted John to a local hospital, under the care of a pediatrician, to discover the underlying problem.

This event occurred in the 1950s when neither CAT scans nor other such sophisticated tests were available. But all the tests that were applicable at the time were carried out in the hospital. The results showed no abnormality. John went home with the diagnosis of "idiopathic convulsive seizures." In medicine, "idiopathic" means "we really don't know."

From that time on, once every week or two the family would awaken me at night with the same scenario. (Fortunately my office was in my home, so I would just throw on a robe.)

All of us were frustrated. Alice, the mother, said, "There must be something wrong with John. It's not normal for a child to have convulsions a couple of times a month like this. Can't you do something?"

My response was, "We performed all the known tests, and we consulted an excellent pediatrician. Nothing turned up any abnormalities. The pediatrician called it 'idiopathic,' which means the cause is unknown."

Anxieties were increasing. I was running out of answers, if I had had any in the first place. I wasn't sure where we could turn. The parents were growing short of patience. Their concern was mounting.

The well-baby examinations and developmental tests, physical and mental, continued to show that the child was normal for his age. I told the mother, "John seems to be gaining weight well. Let him have whole milk now. Stop the formula."

I continued to see him monthly to ease the parents' and my apprehensions. At each visit, I asked about convulsions. Each time his mother would respond excitedly, "He hasn't had any."

He continued to grow and develop normally. The eighth- and ninth-month examinations produced the same response: "John hasn't had more convulsions. Isn't it wonderful? Why did they stop? Should I expect more in the future?"

My answer was, "I don't know. But I would treat him as a normal child and be thankful those dreadful moments have disappeared. I'll treat him as a normal child, also. You don't need to bring him to the office again for a well-baby examination until he is one year old. If you do have any more problems, let me know."

A few months later an article appeared in a medical journal about normal babies with convulsions. The author was a local pediatrician, Dr. David B. Coursin. The conclusions were that a formula in common usage at that time was pyridoxine-deficient. For some babies, this deficiency produced convulsions. John had been drinking this pyridoxine-deficient formula. When he changed to whole milk at six months of age, the convulsive episodes stopped.

That newborn baby had given me an opportunity to achieve medical immortality. I'm sure that I, like all physicians, have had similar opportunities and have failed to discover the cause and the solution. It reminds us to think.

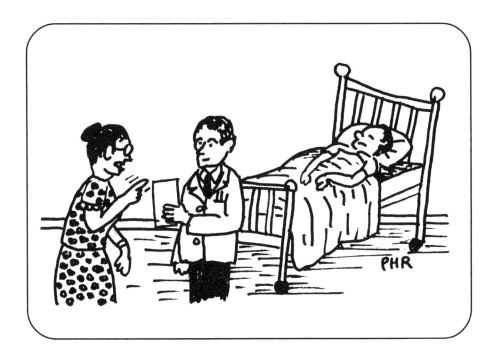

A MIRACLE IN THE 1960S

Concern clouded her voice. Mrs. Albright was telephoning early one morning in the mid-1960s to ask whether I could stop by to see her husband, Arthur.

While at an ice hockey game the previous evening, he had developed pain in his chest. He drove home and, not wanting to bother his family doctor with what after all might be "nothing more than indigestion," had endured his recurring pain through the night. Still suffering when daybreak occurred, he at last agreed to let his wife call me. I told her I would come over at once.

As I talked with the 56-year-old man and examined him, I quickly concluded that he had suffered a myocardial infarction. We called an ambulance to take him to the Lancaster General Hospital. (There were no emergency medical technicians at that time.)

Arthur entered a medical intensive care unit, comprising a four-bed ward with two cardiac monitors. This unit had been established just a few months previously. I had given him morphine sulfate at home. Shortly after he arrived at the hospital, a staff nurse noted that his blood pressure was low. We started an intravenous drip with Levophed medication, a vasopressor, to attempt to maintain his systolic blood pressure over 90 millimeters of mercury. I had notified consultants as soon as he was admitted, and together we initiated procedures appropriate for a recent coronary occlusion. In those days, care involved pain relief, monitoring blood pressure and rhythm for any irregularities and observing for any signs of congestive heart failure.

An electrocardiogram showed evidence of an extensive anterior myocardial infarction. Enzyme studies were not yet available.

We informed his wife of his guarded prognosis. They had a son who lived at home. And they had a daughter, a registered nurse— a graduate of the Lancaster General Hospital School of Nursing, in fact—who was a missionary in a Third World country in Africa. Her mother notified their daughter, Ruth, of her father's serious illness and she made plans to fly home within a few days.

At that time and place we could offer no alternative to good medical care. Heart surgery and other invasive procedures were simply not available. After 48 hours, we made an attempt to gradually decrease the rate of flow of the Levophed medication, with the hope that Arthur's blood pressure would be maintained. We found that every decrease in the medication resulted in a decrease in his blood pressure. As a result, we resumed the infusion at the original rate.

After ten days of continuous treatment with the Levophed intravenous drip, the cardiologists thought that we should again try decreasing the rate. They wanted to see whether his cardiovascular system could respond and stabilize his blood pressure.

By this time Ruth had arrived home. I had explained his condition to his wife and obtained her consent to proceed with this recommendation. But now I received a major surprise. When I talked with his daughter about the problem, her response was, "Oh, you're trying to play God. I can't permit you to do that."

I said, "Your father has had an extensive myocardial infarction. A large part of his heart muscle is unable to function. With a vasopressor medication, the cardiologists have been able to achieve adequate blood pressure to maintain his circulation. But we cannot continue the medication forever. Your father deserves a better quality of life than that. At some point, we must reduce the amount of vasopressor he's receiving to see whether his heart and blood vessels can respond satisfactorily." She seemed unconvinced.

When I explained Ruth's reaction to the consultants, they replied, "We can't stop the medication if she feels that way." The treatment was continued and the patient continued to do well.

A week passed. Arthur's daughter remained solemn and thoughtful. One day she said to me, "We can't continue this indefinitely. I don't want Dad to be kept a prisoner by an intravenous line the rest of his life. What should we do?"

"What would you like us to do, Ruth?"

"I guess you can tell the consultants to decrease the medication and see what happens."

"You realize he may not be able to maintain an adequate blood pressure and circulation without the medicine." I hesitated a moment. "He may die."

"I've discussed our predicament with my mother and brother. All of us agree. We must try."

We gradually decreased the Levophed flow rate. Then, 48 hours later, we discontinued this medication. It was somewhat risky, we knew. I thought it possible that I could receive a call anytime during the night.

Imagine my astonishment when I entered Arthur's room the next morning. He sat up in bed and said, "Great to see you, Dr. Wentz!"

I said, "How are you feeling?"

"I'm fine."

After an additional two weeks of hospitalization, Arthur went home. His systolic blood pressure never exceeded 94 and was frequently in the mid 80s. This meant that his activity was severely limited. But his mind had remained clear throughout his illness.

He survived about six months. Congestive heart failure would no longer respond to medical treatment. Too much heart muscle had been damaged.

But through a miracle I still don't fully comprehend, Arthur Albright had been granted an additional half year to spend with his family.

In more recent times, patients and their families have been educated to seek medical attention promptly for chest pain. Physicians have been trained to get the victim to the hospital immediately with the help of trained medical personnel. Hopefully, heart muscle can be saved.

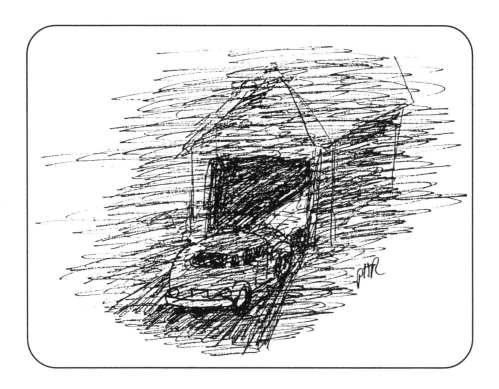

FOG IN A COVERED BRIDGE

I had the privilege of caring for a woman who was 103 years old. In recent months Susan Bolder had been moved from her home in Strasburg to a nursing home about seven miles away. I regularly continued to visit her in her new surroundings. She had developed heart failure, and now she was taking the appropriate medications and eating a low-salt diet.

At 2:15 a.m. the telephone rang. "Can you come to see Susie Bolder?"

"What's the trouble?"

"She seems short of breath and is unable to rest. We've been giving her oxygen."

"I'll be there."

Quickly I dressed and got into my car. As I exited the garage, I became aware of impaired vision because of a heavy fog. In the village of Strasburg, driving was relatively easy because buildings were close to the road on both sides and I could see their images through the fog. But as soon as I got out of town, I could see only the white line in the middle of the road. This was in the 1950s, prior to the time white lines were painted on both sides of the road. I followed the center white line. At 2:30 a.m. there was no traffic on the road. My journey took me over a covered bridge. As I approached it, I could follow the center white line on the road with no difficulty. But in the bridge itself there was no white line. I was unable to see either side or the other end of the bridge. I rolled down the window of my car and stretched out my arm seeking the left side of the bridge with my fingers. As I drove straight ahead, my fingers guided me through the bridge. It was fortunate that there was no traffic, for I crossed a major highway, Route 30, without seeing it. Finally, I arrived at the nursing home.

Even with the oxygen mask over her face, Susie was in obvious distress with labored breathing. Her pulse rate was rapid but the rhythm was regular. Blood pressure was satisfactory. I examined her heart and lungs. Her heart was enlarged. She had rales in her lungs indicating pulmonary congestion secondary to heart failure. I administered a diuretic and a sedative by injection. We discussed the option of hospitalization which she rejected. (This was prior to Medicare.) I considered her age of 103 and did not dispute her decision. In a short time she was breathing easier and resting more comfortably.

I drove home the same way I had come, using the same method to cross the covered bridge. I was happy to return safely, content that I had helped an elderly woman live peaceably a while longer as I crawled into bed for a little more sleep.

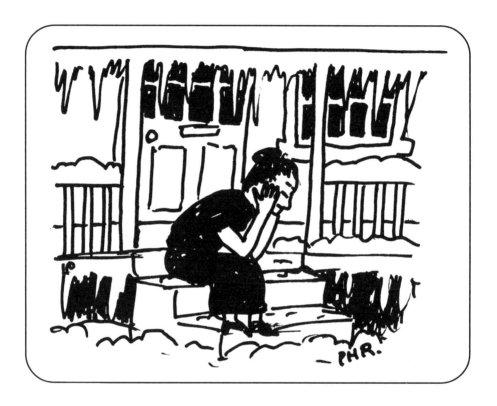

COMPETENT OR INCOMPETENT

Mrs. Nellie Irons, in her middle eighties, owned a considerable portion of land. She was a widow with no children.

I had cared for her husband until he died, and I continued to provide medical care for her. She had borderline cardiac failure, requiring digitalization and diuretics along with a low-salt diet and considerable rest.

On recent visits I had become concerned about her mental clarity and ability to take medicine correctly. She lived alone, and her closest relative was a niece whom I had never met.

On April 11, I recorded my concerns about her ability to take her medicine properly and listed several references to backup my suspicions. On a cold December day the previous year, a concerned neighbor had called me because she was sitting on a stoop on her back porch. I went to her home. Despite the temperature, she had had only a shawl over her shoulders. Her hands were cold, cold, cold. I took her inside the house and stood her in front of the coal range to get warm. She didn't seem to know why she had been sitting outside.

During my more recent visits, I'd found that she had more medicine remaining than I thought there should be. (When I dispensed medicine, usually the amounts given coincided with the time between her scheduled visits.) At times her answers did not seem relevant to my questions. Now, as I recorded my observations, I also noted that I had decided to call her niece to express my concerns.

About four months later Ed, a lawyer and a fraternity brother with whom I had gone to college, called to tell me that Nellie Irons had sold the same piece of property twice in recent months. The court had scheduled a hearing to evaluate her competency. I believe that he wanted to prove her soundness of mind. He intended to demonstrate that real estate agents had confused her or provided unreliable information and that this had led her to sell the same property two times.

In days to come, Ed would see me on the street and chide me, "Henry, you'd better be prepared for Nellie's hearing. You're going to come off looking bad if you attempt to show that she's incompetent." Another time he said, "I'm going to get you when I get you in court." I never told him about the notes I had on Nellie's records about her loss of mental faculties.

The day arrived in October. All of us appeared in court. Ed explained to the judge the reasons for the hearing and said that he was prepared to prove Mrs. Irons competent on the day of the first sale in May.

My time arrived. I was called to the witness stand and sworn in.

"Dr. Wentz, do you know Mrs. Nellie Irons?"

"Yes."

"How do you know her?"

"I have been her physician for the last 12 years."

"Do you have any reason according to your professional judgment to consider this woman incompetent?"

I took out my records and started to read, "On April 11 of this year, I wrote the following notes into the medical records of Mrs. Nellie Irons: 'For several months I have been concerned about her mental clarity. In December of last year, I was called and informed that she was sitting outside the back door of her home on a stoop on a bitter cold winter day. When I visited her sitting there, she seemed to be in a daze or trance and not well oriented about her surroundings. Although she says that she takes her medicine regularly according to instructions, there was, on an office visit, too much medicine remaining in her medicine envelopes to substantiate her statement.' I dispense my own medicine and know how much she has been given. I ask my patients to bring their medicine with them, so I can verify their compliance and answer any questions about their medication."

I continued to read from my records, "'I am concerned that she is not taking her medicine correctly because of some loss of her mental faculties and am troubled that she may run into serious problems from either taking too much or not enough of her medications. I will call her niece to express my concerns and will get information from her about what we should do.'"

These words from my records seemed to set the tone of the hearing. I was told some time later that the judge had declared Nellie Irons incompetent. I was never made aware of the legal implications that followed. My lawyer friend, Ed, never said another word to me about Mrs. Irons.

The lesson to be learned from this story is the importance of keeping records on a patient's mental state as well as physical condition.

MARRIED FOR LOVE

In the early 1950s, my only office assistant was my wife, Mary. She did my bookkeeping, paid the bills, and sent the bills to patients. She also helped me in the office when I needed help with a female patient.

One afternoon I was seeing a young woman for a neighboring physician, who was on a vacation. This patient said, "I'm pregnant, and I haven't been able to keep anything in my stomach, not even water, for the last three days."

Her husband, who had accompanied her, was holding her hand and appeared very sympathetic. He echoed her remarks: "Doc, she hasn't kept anything down for at least two days. I'm worried about her and the baby."

I tried to reassure both of them. She did not seem dehydrated. Her vital signs were good; and, when I compared the weight they had given me at her doctor's office from a week before, I found that her weight at my office was about the same. Maybe she now weighed a pound less.

At that time, it was customary to emphasize diet with frequent small feedings and to give vitamin B-6 (pyridoxine) intravenous injections from one to three times a week for nausea and vomiting due to pregnancy. I had gone over a printed diet with this young woman, and now I prepared an injection. I had decided that, because she was another physician's patient and did not have other complaints, I would not examine her further at that time.

I drew 100 milligrams of pyridoxine into a sterile syringe from a multiple-dose vial. I used a blood pressure cuff as a tourniquet and prepared to give the injection. Her husband held her hand more tightly and leaned solicitously over her, saying, "It won't hurt a bit, Sweetheart. It will be over in a minute, Dearie. Be brave! This will help you and our baby, Sweetie."

The injection went forward without further incident. After paying me for the visit and medication, the patient and her husband left the office.

A few minutes later, I heard a sharp knock on the door. The husband burst in crying, "My wife passed out in the car!"

"Please bring her into the office again. I'll examine her."

By the time she came back into the office, she seemed alert and in good condition. Her vital signs were unchanged. Her blood pressure was in the 90s, as it previously had been, and that was not unusual in early pregnancy. I took more history, inquiring about her menstrual cycle, her last period, any vaginal bleeding, and any abdominal pain or discomfort. All answers were negative except for her comments about the extreme nausea and vomiting she had undergone. I said, "I want to examine you, including a check of your abdomen and pelvis, to make sure things are all right. My wife will come in to help you get ready and will stay with you during the examination."

I called Mary into the office, then I stepped out until everything was ready. Mary called me back into the office, and I completed the examination without finding anything unusual. She was in early pregnancy, but no other problems were evident. After she dressed, I again reassured her and her husband that everything was all right and dismissed them from the office. I thought the syncopal episode, or whatever it had been, was a sympathetic reaction to the injection.

After they had driven away, Mary said, "Do you know what that young lady asked me?"

"No."

"She asked me whether I was a nurse. I told her that I was not, but that I was only helping my husband in the office. She then told me that she thought all doctors married nurses. And then she said, 'Then you married for love!'"

I could hardly wait until my neighboring physician returned from vacation to tell him that story. Why? Because he had married a nurse!

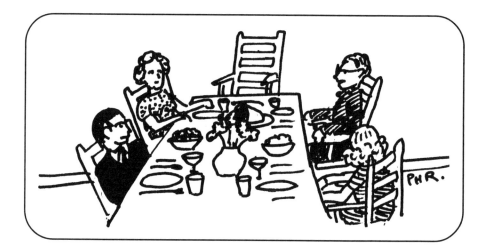

AN EVENING TO REMEMBER

One evening we were looking forward to a special event in our lives. Our son, Bill, was going to bring his girlfriend to our house for dinner.

Mary, my wife, had informed me, "I expect you to be home the entire time. I want you to offer the blessing, carve the meat and make conversation until they leave."

The house was in order for company. We had all showered and dressed in our best Sunday clothing to await their arrival. There were Mother and Dad and Bill's sister, Louise, about ten years old.

Bill arrived with Gloria, a very pretty teenager with blue eyes and natural blonde hair. She lived in a small town about eight miles from Strasburg. Mary called us to dinner. We sat down to a beautifully decorated table and the aroma of beef and peas and a fresh salad.

"We thank you, O God for this food. Give us grateful and joyful hearts...."

A loud vibrating buzzer sounded, interrupting everything. Living in the house with my medical office on the lower level, all of us except Gloria were aware that this was the emergency buzzer in the office. Its sound, petrifying in its intensity, was the patient's way of getting our attention. It did not always signify an emergency. Somebody could be calling for medicine. Somebody could want a form or paper they had left at the office, or want an appointment, or even wish to pay a bill. There were many things for which a person might want to get our attention. Since my wife had said, "You be there," and all schedules had been arranged for this occasion, I said, "Louise, will you please go down to the office and see what that person wants?"

I began to carve the meat. Within two minutes we heard Louise running up the stairs and screaming for Mother and Daddy, "Janine's grandfather is here and bleeding from every place there is! I let him in, and blood's all over the walls and floor!"

I bolted from the room, throwing down my napkin and not even asking our guest to excuse me.

Bill Miller was a prominent man in this small town of Strasburg. Further, he was the father of one of our friends and the grandfather of Janine, one of Louise's classmates and best friends.

Louise had not exaggerated. There was blood everywhere. In fact, with blood all over Bill's face and hair, I found it at first difficult to recognize him. I got him into an examining room, laid him on a table and saw that his left ear was almost severed from his head. He was bleeding profusely from an open artery in that area. With my best clothes on, I seized a hemostat and clamped the artery to stop the bleeding, only to see that blood was coming from several other places on the scalp and face.

In clamping the artery I had pointed the spurting blood in my direction so my jacket and trousers were sprayed. At this point, belatedly, I took off my jacket, placed a plastic apron over my clothing and sought other bleeding points, as well as trying to see what portions of Bill's anatomy had been lacerated. The large part of his left external ear was just hanging there by some skin. The other lacerations were bleeding and open, but not as severe. Blood was spread over his arms and clothing. I tried to determine whether other parts of the body were injured or if the blood was all from the head wounds.

As I prepared to take his blood pressure and his pulse (nobody else was on hand and I thought I could not ask somebody upstairs to help), I began to evaluate what I was going to do. Clearly, Bill Miller had to go to the hospital. But I hardly could take the time away from more important procedures to call for help. His blood pressure was barely obtainable from all the loss of blood, and his pulse was rapid and thready. I ran to another room to get an intravenous solution, which would improve his fluid volume, and decided that as soon as that was started and running satisfactorily, I would take the time to call the local ambulance.

By this time, most of the bleeding was controlled; but there were a few dangling hemostats, as I hadn't taken the time to put ligatures in place.

As usual when one is in a hurry, nothing goes well. With the blood pressure down, I had difficulty placing the needle in the vein; that caused delay. This was in the days before modern intravenous gadgets were available. I was using an ordinary needle, praying that it would stay in place. Finally—it seemed like hours instead of minutes—the fluid was running into his vascular system.

I called for the local ambulance explaining, "I have an accident emergency with a lot of blood loss. I'm all alone and need some help. This is an emergency. Please come at once!"

Now I took the time to inquire what had happened. He said, "I ran into an Amish horse and buggy at an intersection just outside Strasburg when the buggy suddenly turned left in front of me. The windshield broke and cut me. Somebody—I don't know who—picked me up and brought me over here."

I said, "You lost a lot of blood. I started some intravenous fluid. You'll have to go...." I was interrupted by a convulsion as Bill jerked and quivered all over. I ran again to get oxygen. I figured this seizure was the result of blood loss, decreased blood pressure and circulation, and an inadequate supply of oxygen to his brain. It could have been from the head injury or some other problems as yet undiagnosed. Since I could not do anything about the other problems at the moment, I looked at the IV to assure myself it was running, opened the clamp wide to increase the flow into his vascular system, said a little prayer with my eyes wide open, and elatedly watched as stillness came over his body. A few seconds later he was asking, "What happened?"

I watched him closely and started to attend to his wounds. First I applied ligatures to the arteries so I could remove the hemostats. I told him, "I think you lost a little too much blood, and that caused you to black out for a short time."

His blood pressure had been up a little during the seizure and now was in the 90s which represented an improvement.

And now we heard the most reassuring sound: the ambulance was finally approaching. I had gotten a few sutures in place to hold Bill's ear in position. I opened the office door and welcomed the ambulance attendants. I asked them to help me put on a pressure dressing around his head to stop the oozing and hold the ear in place. Then we transferred him from the examining table to a litter. I had strapped his arm to a board and taped over the needle to keep it in place. I held the bottle and asked for another that I could add en route to the hospital. Preoccupied, I had temporarily forgotten the party upstairs. Now I realized I must let the others know that I was going along to the hospital and would not be returning for a few hours.

Unfortunately in those days ambulance attendants were not trained except in the necessary rudiments of first aid. So I needed to accompany this unstable patient in the ambulance, monitor his vital signs, make certain the IV kept running, change bottles if necessary, be ready for more convulsive episodes, and have a surgeon see him at the hospital.

There were no specially trained emergency room physicians. After the patient was in the ambulance I took time over the inter-communications system we had in the house and office to buzz my wife: "I'll be going with Mr. Miller in the ambulance and may not be back for a couple of hours. Please call the Lancaster General Hospital emergency room, tell them we're on our way, and have a surgeon meet us there." Ambulances had no two-way radios or methods of communicating with the hospital, so I had to ask Mary to do it for us.

I hung up the phone as my wife was asking, "What shall I do with your...?"

I hurriedly climbed into the back of the ambulance beside the patient. Again I checked his blood pressure and pulse, asking, "How are you feeling?"

His blood pressure now was over 100, and I felt somewhat relieved when he replied, "Not bad. I have a headache."

I told the driver, "Put on the siren. Go as fast as you can go safely. Don't go through intersections without slowing down. I don't have any idea what his blood count is but I know he needs blood, and this fluid will have to do until we can get some." I continued to administer oxygen as we hastened along our way for the ten-mile ride to the hospital.

A surgeon met us at the emergency room. As soon as I had communicated to the surgeon about the multiple extensive lacerations with considerable blood loss and initial unstable vital signs, I said, "You are in good hands. The surgeon will take good care of you. I'll see you to-morrow when you're feeling better. Bye!" Immediately I got the ambulance crew together for our return to Strasburg.

The party was over. Gloria and Bill had gone. Louise was still upset at this blood-curdling experience of seeing her friend's grandfather in this condition. She did not sleep well that night. And I had to face my wife, who had had to assume all of the responsibility for entertaining on that special occasion. "What do you mean leaving me alone with Bill and his friend with a dinner to serve? Did you really have to go along with the ambulance? Why didn't you tell me what to expect when you called me over the intercom before you went to the hospital with the ambulance, instead of hanging up in my ear in the middle of a question?"

"Bill's condition was unstable, and he could have died on the way to the hospital. I had to go along. I didn't know what to expect, so I couldn't very well tell you. We were in such a hurry I couldn't take the time for a longer conversation."

"I'll never plan another dinner party for the family or anybody else. I can't go on with all these interruptions in our lives. There must be a way to avoid these situations if you really want to."

"I don't like this any better than you do. I was looking forward to this event, too. You must admit this was unusual."

And so to bed with both of us tired, frustrated and angry. When Bill returned, I said, "I'm sorry."

He said, "I understand, Dad."

Neither of our children entered the field of medicine for a career. Could this and other negative experiences in the family have influenced their decision?

A few months later, I enrolled in a day-long postgraduate course for general practitioners at Temple University. While the doctors were learning about new and up-to-date procedures, a university psychiatrist rounded up our wives to discuss what it was like to be a physician's wife and any stresses they wished to share. After several wives had sounded off about their problems, Mary told this story and the way a physician's family differs from others. The psychiatrist exploded: "I never heard anything so ridiculous. When a doctor has a special evening, nothing should be allowed to interrupt him. What do you mean? Sending a ten-year-old girl to an emergency!"

Mary said, "What else could he have done? Let him bleed to death? Who would have taken care of him? There are many people who use that buzzer for things other than emergencies. When we sent Louise we didn't realize what a scene she would encounter."

The psychiatrist said, "When you plan a special evening, you should arrange to have another physician take your calls. Your evening should not be interrupted. You should never send a ten-year-old to see what the emergency is."

"We did have another doctor taking calls. But he was not at our office and this patient did not call so we could refer him to another doctor. He just arrived unannounced."

Mary was getting nowhere, so she said, "It's easy for you to sit in your 'Ivory Tower' and tell people what to do. You have never been out in a rural area with a situation like this." This psychiatrist would never understand the problems of a small-town physician just as we could not understand the situations he might meet in the big city.

After the conference, though, she did let me know how over dedicated I was to my practice and that we should be able to make some changes to reduce the demands on our lives and the lives of our children. She summarized her viewpoint and feelings this way: "We should never send one of our children to the emergency door in the future. This situation seemed unavoidable and was unusual. If a similar situation should arise again, your responsibilities and actions would have to be the same. We should continue to plan our free time and have other physicians take our calls. And we should leave the house, so we will not be there for any unannounced arrivals."

Today most people go to hospital emergency rooms for accidents, and ambulance attendants are well-trained. As a result of these improvements in medical care for patients who have experienced trauma and other emergencies, physicians are much less likely to have such "an evening to remember."

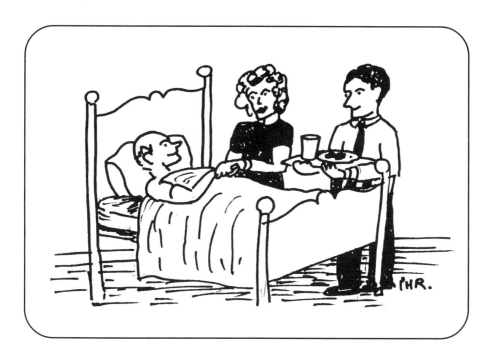

THERE'S NO PLACE LIKE HOME

"I hate the hospital."

These were the words of John, a 75-year-old-man who had been hospitalized numerous times for a failing heart. He had voiced this comment repeatedly before, during and after his last few hospital admissions.

At the time of his latest admission, John realized he would never recover. He told his son-in-law, "You may as well sell my car. I won't be needing it anymore."

His last admission had been for heart failure and increasing retention of fluid in his abdomen, legs and lungs. We had prescribed oxygen, a low-salt diet, increased use of diuretics and rest. John's frequent question was, "Why can't I die at home?"

He had been in the hospital so often for the same reason that he knew the routine by heart. But that didn't make it any easier. John kept thinking that with help he could have better "comfort care" at home. Sometimes he wasn't bathed until late in the morning or worse, was left in the middle of a bath because a nurse had something more urgent to do. It was difficult for Virginia, his wife, to get to the hospital. She didn't drive and was a partial invalid herself, with poor eyesight, diabetes and arthritis that caused some difficulty in getting around. The low-salt diet wasn't appetizing; he knew he needed that, but maybe he could have more things he liked without salt. He knew laboratory tests were to be done frequently to check on electrolytes and renal function, among other things because of his need for strong diuretics. He needed to closely follow the directions for his heart medicine. His condition called for an occasional chest x-ray. But all of this could be arranged at home with a proper support system. By this time he had been a patient in the hospital for more than six weeks.

Jean, the only child of John and his wife, was a nurse who had a full-time job in a physician's office. She had a husband and two teenage boys at home. "I can get a nurse at night so Mom can get a good night's sleep," she told me as her parents listened. "The nurse can bathe him in the morning and get him cleaned up before she goes. Mom can get breakfast and spend the morning with him. My husband, Jim, can come for lunch. A nurse can be with him a few hours in the late afternoon and can prepare dinner for both of them, and Jim and I can visit in the evening. The family doctor can see him at home as needed."

Her mother smiled and said, "That would be great. I could really do more than that."

"No, Mom. We're trying to keep him at home. If you get too tired and don't get your rest, our plans will go to pieces."

"Well, all right."

"How do you feel about that, Dad?" Jean asked. "Remember, it may not always be the optimum in medical treatment at home, and you may be uncomfortable and in distress at times. But we'll do our best to help you. All things must come to an end sometime, but we will allow the end to come at home if that is what you want."

"It sounds good to me. I don't want to come back to this place. They take care of me very well, but there is no place like home."

Together the family members and I set in motion actions to implement the plan. When the optimum in his hospital treatment had been reached, John was discharged.

He left the hospital after lunch one day and went home by ambulance. A hospital bed, oxygen, a bedside commode and other needed supplies were already there. A woman came about 3:30 p.m. to take care of his needs. She prepared dinner for Mom and Pop and left after they had eaten. Jean arrived with her husband and administered to John's needs, while Jim went to the pharmacy for John's medicine. Another nurse came and stayed with him during the night and, in addition, gave Virginia, John's wife, peace of mind so she could rest. The nurse gave John his morning care and started his breakfast before she left. As his physician, I stopped by a few days later to check on John and to see how everything was progressing.

He said, "I feel fine. How much do I need this oxygen?"

I said, "You are doing well. Use the oxygen as you feel you need it for shortness of breath. I'll set it for you and all anybody has to do is turn it on when you want it. I turned to Virginia. "How are you doing, Mom?"

"I'm getting along fine."

"Be sure you follow the diet for John, and you get plenty of rest when other help is here."

Jim, John's son-in-law, had a full-time job at an industrial plant about a mile and a half from his father-in-law's home. Every weekday at 11:45 a.m. Jim would arrive. "How are things going?" he asked John one day.

"I'm feeling a little down today. I had a miserable cough last night and Mom was up a lot, and neither of us slept so well. Do you think I should go back to the hospital?"

"You're the one to decide that. Remember, you never wanted to go back. You said you'd rather ride it out at home."

"I know, but we didn't sleep so well last night. Mom will tire out."

"Well, let's try to help you. Jean will be in tonight. Maybe she'll have a few suggestions. Maybe you could use the oxygen more at night. Let's eat lunch."

They would all eat lunch together, John and Mom and Jim, and talk. John said to Jim, "I know I'm not going to get any better. Why can't I die?"

Jim replied, "You've had this problem a long time. I guess you and all of us must learn to live with it. Some days will be good and some not so good, but we'll all try to support and help you in any way we can. Do you want anything before I leave? Let's take a little walk around these two rooms."

Answering John's repeated question, "Why can't I die?" was probably the most difficult part of the entire situation.

Jim helped John out of bed and around the rooms, then to the commode and back to bed. "Jean and I'll be in to see you this evening."

When they arrived each evening, dinner would be over. Jean would wash the dishes and clean up a little while Jim would run any needed errands to get medicine or food.

John said to Jean, "I guess Jim told you we didn't have such a good night last night."

"Yes. Did you get short of breath? Are you passing a good bit of urine? Can you reach the urinal okay?"

"I was a little short of breath. Not too bad. But the cough bothered me. I pass a good bit of urine."

"Take a rest pill tonight and stay propped up in bed. Use your oxygen. See how that goes. If you continue to have trouble, we'll have the doctor see you again. Is Mom sticking to your low-salt diet? Jim said you were talking about going back to the hospital again. Do you really mean that? Are you getting scared?"

"Yeah. I mentioned it. I don't want to tire Mother. Jim made me feel better about it. I don't want to go back. I just don't want to make it too difficult for everybody."

"You're doing okay. We'll help you. Let the night nurse help you." Then she turned to Mom and continued, "Mom, let the nurse take care of him. That is why she is here. You rest. The nurse will call you if she needs you."

Mom said, "I'll try. It's a lot easier having him here than running back and forth to the hospital when it's so difficult to get there. I don't drive, so I have to depend on somebody else."

The support system worked well at home. Laboratory technicians came and took blood when tests were necessary. The nurses did a good job. But John leaned on Jim for his emotional and physical support. He looked forward to their luncheon dates, when he and Mom and Jim were alone and he could ask his son-in-law all his questions and tell him his troubles.

"How are things today?"

"I'd like to take a little walk around the room. I'm getting tired of just sitting or lying in bed. Maybe I could sit in that chair over there to eat lunch and then you can put me back in bed before you go."

"Okay. Here we go." He uncovered John, stood him up, placed a robe on him and took his arm for a walk around a very small room. Then he put a fluffy cushion on the stuffed chair and helped him sit down. He brought John his tray, placed it on a small table in front of his chair, cut his meat, buttered his bread and helped him feed himself. "Is it good?"

"I guess as good as you can expect without salt. It feels good to be out here for a while."

On another occasion John was feeling down. He said to Jim, "Why can't I die? Why can't death be made easier? Last night I could hardly get my breath. After a difficult time, the nurse gave me a shot. After a long time, it felt like an hour, I finally went to sleep. When I woke up this morning, I felt better. Do you think I should go to the hospital? Could they do more for me?"

"I guess they could do a little more. Could they keep you more comfortable? I don't know. You've been there a number of times. What do you think? It was your decision to stay home. But we can always do something different if you change your mind. I guess it boils down to the question, Do you want to die in the hospital or at home? Can we help you adequately at home?"

"Maybe I could just sleep away after one of those shots. Wouldn't that be wonderful? I'd rather be home."

One day several weeks later when Jim arrived, John said, "Who are you? Why are you here?"

"I'm here to have lunch with you," Jim said. "I'm Jim, Jean's husband. Don't you remember?"

"Where's Mom?"

"Right here in her chair."

"No. I mean my mother. I don't mean my wife. I want my mother."

"We'll help you. What would you like us to do?"

As his condition deteriorated, John's mind became more confused. There were bad days and good days. He became combative and uncooperative when he was not in control of his senses. It got more difficult for all care-givers, especially Mom, whom he seemed to fight the most. Jim seemed to be able to help calm him and not confront him with his confusion and mistakes. He would change his wet bed and clothes, feed him, listen to him and offer help.

And one day death arrived.

I came in and pronounced him dead as the family gathered around. Although death came not unexpectedly and almost as a blessing, its finality caused weeping and sadness to overflow.

"He got his wish. He died at home, and I think we were able to keep him fairly comfortable," said Jean.

"Yes. I'm glad," Mom said between sobs, "I could help take care of him here, and the nurses were so helpful."

"When he was aware, he seemed happy and satisfied here. Everybody did a good job," Jim said.

When death came to John, all involved with his last days were aware that his devoted family had spent many hours in caring for him during the preceding six to eight months and that this concern and attention had not been in vain. Caring had contributed to his well-being and comfort and, most of all, to his peace of mind.

In particular, a devoted son-in-law had contributed greatly to his terminal care.

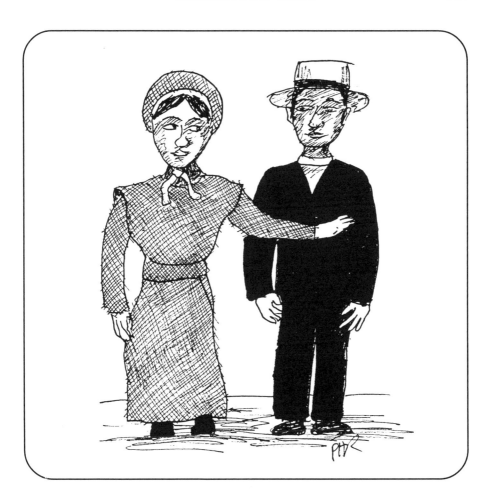

EXPERIENCE

BEGETS BEHAVIOR

Paul had had a heart attack. In the 1960s he had recovered from a posterior coronary artery occlusion, which was considered less life-threatening than occlusion of an anterior coronary artery. In those days patients with serious heart conditions were normally kept in the hospital at least 21 days, then spent one month of relative rest at home. During the third month the patient who had no complications was encouraged to gradually return to normal activity in anticipation of a return to work.

Paul had had an uncomplicated convalescence, and I had full intentions of gradually increasing his activities. I anticipated that, without any unexpected problems, he would be able to return to his work as a clerk in a hardware store at the beginning of the fourth month following his heart attack.

I saw him in the office every two weeks. Every time his wife, Anna, accompanied him. I always appreciated the spouse's being involved with her husband's medical care. But Anna seemed different. On each visit, I asked him about his activity: "Have you been going up or down steps more than once a day? Have you been walking out-of-doors? Have you been driving the car?"

Anna would always answer for him: "Yes, he's been doing that."

Paul would look a little perplexed, then offer, "She says I've been doing that, but really I've been doing very little."

"Why haven't you been doing those things? Don't you feel well? Are you having some problems?"

They'd look at each other, then Anna would say, "We'll try to do better next time."

As I tried to analyze the situation, I got the impression it was Anna who was holding him back, not permitting him to progress to the next step.

Each visit seemed a repeat of the previous one, and I became increasingly frustrated. I tried to explain to both of them the need for accelerating the pace of Paul's exercising. I wanted my goal to be their goal; namely, to return him to work at the end of three months.

The resistance continued, and the negative response seemed to be led by his wife. I couldn't understand her protective behavior.

At one time I thought that this reluctance might be a personal thing, a lack of confidence in me or a personal negative feeling toward me. I suggested having Paul see a consultant to assure both of them of his good recovery and to encourage increased activities. After my continued suggestions, they accepted this idea and saw a cardiologist. He did provide reassurance and gave specific recommendations.

Still the inactivity continued, and whatever progress was made was slow. I felt myself getting more and more frustrated. I saw the goal of returning to work being stretched to four months, even six months or longer. He was being turned into a helpless, dependent invalid; I felt that in this way they were just increasing Paul's risk of further cardiac problems. He was getting little exercise, and he would soon develop an attitude suggesting that life as he had known it was over.

Paul and Anna were Reformed Mennonites. He dressed in a dark suit with a Nehru-like collar, with either no tie or a black bowtie, and wore either a straw or black broad-brimmed hat. Anna was dressed in a full-length gray dress with a cape of the same color. She wore a head covering under a large gray bonnet. I felt quite certain that their religion played no part in this behavior toward Paul's convalescence.

And then came the revelation!

One day Anna made an appointment for a physical examination. I took a family history. Her father had died of a heart attack;

her mother had died of a heart attack; her two brothers had died of heart attacks; one sister had died of a heart attack; some grandparents had died of heart attacks.

Now I finally understood. To Anna, heart attack meant death. No wonder she protected her husband. No wonder she never let him out of her sight. She wanted him around for a while. She did not want to be a widow.

For the first time I understood Anna's protective behavior, her reluctance to allow him to work, her rejection of my suggestions. My frustration changed into a challenge.

Now I could relate to her feelings. Now I could work with her, recognizing her anxieties and fears. I addressed these. I talked with Paul and Anna and with much reassurance was able to return Paul to full-time work in five months. And I believe she allowed him to live a fairly normal life, although occasionally some of Anna's protectiveness again reared its head!

It was easy to see how Anna's experiences with heart attacks in her family had influenced her behavior. After all of us realized the problem, we could work together.

And I'm happy to be able to report that Paul led a happy and productive life for years afterward.

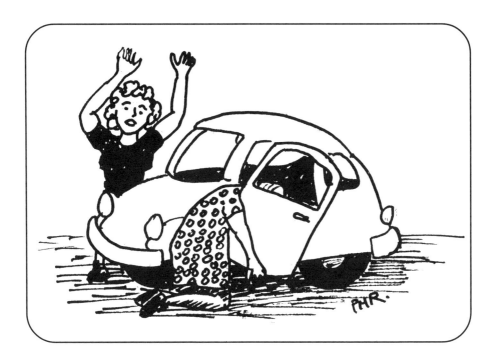

SAVED BY A SCREAM

A neighboring physician, Dr. Krusen, was on vacation.

One bright July afternoon in the 1960s a young mother, a patient of his whom I had never seen before, brought her five-year-old daughter to my office. The daughter had cut her hand opening a can of soup. Her laceration required stitches.

It was a day on which I did not have office hours, so I had to do everything myself. I got everything ready to repair the tear in her skin. Then I cleansed the wound with copious amounts of soap and water and painted the entire area with Betadyne solution.

I put on sterile gloves and placed over the wound a drape with a hole in the center. I had already opened a sterile pack containing the instruments I'd need, along with gauze, suture material and local anesthetic. I injected xylocaine around the wound to numb the area. Then I began placing sutures in the laceration to draw together the edges of the wound.

I was busily occupied with this repair when the mother said, "I think I'll go outside while you finish working on Jean."

I said, "Okay," and proceeded with my job, tying knots in the sutures and cutting the ends.

Suddenly, I heard a scream outside. Dropping the instruments, I flung open the emergency door that opened to the outside and the parking lot. I saw Jean's mother hanging from the door of her Volkswagen. She had opened the door to get in and apparently had fainted. As her body collapsed, her neck had wedged in the space between the door and the frame of the car. Now she was hanging there, choking. I ran to her assistance, picked her up—fortunately, she was not a heavy woman—and laid her down on the macadam parking lot as she began to respond from her life-threatening fall. The scream had come from an older daughter, who had remained outside when her mother brought her sister into the office for medical care.

The main lesson I learned from this experience is that whenever I detect that a person doesn't feel normal and wants to go into another room or to step outside for fresh air, I should insist that he or she lie down on the floor where I can keep an eye on everything.

How fortunate it was that another daughter had remained outside with the car!

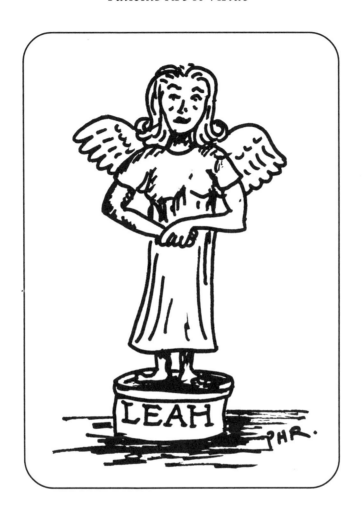

THE WILL TO CHANGE

Fred Ireland was about 50 years old when I first met him in my office. The manager of a local business, he was complaining of backache. Studies of his back showed much to create his discomfort. With exercises and medication and care of his back, he seemed able to live with it in relative comfort.

After I had seen him for a few years, off and on, Fred came in one day with a different complaint: a backache that was a little different and some vague indigestion. He was now in his late 50s, of average height and stocky build. He was a likable man, understandably concerned about his health. He smiled but little as he related his complaints.

A concern of some serious underlying problem, which is the way a doctor is trained and something we are always thinking about, made me evaluate his complaints for some new disorder. After x-rays and blood tests (ultrasound was not yet available) my suspicion of pancreatic cancer was not confirmed. But I suspected it even more intensely.

As I thought about this early diagnosis, before jaundice and other physical signs and symptoms developed, I made arrangements for his admission to the hospital in a few days. He needed time to get his affairs in order at work and at home, as he would be absent for several weeks.

Fred lived with his family on a small farm. His wife, Leah, worked in a clerical position. They had a 10-year-old daughter, Jean.

Unfortunately, by the time he was admitted to the hospital jaundice was in evidence. Tests confirmed my preliminary diagnosis. Fred underwent palliative surgery.

He came home, worked as he was able and took medicine for mitigation of pain. Eventually he was confined to his home. His wife, Leah, took excellent care of him, kept him comfortable and gave him a lot of emotional support. Finally, he succumbed to his illness.

Fred's father, Harry, lived alone about 20 miles away. He had been estranged from his wife, Fred's mother, for almost a quarter century. Harry had been a successful businessman and had retired to a small house in the woods several miles north of Lancaster. He had always been self-sufficient and had spent little time with his son and his family.

Fred had brought his father to see me several years before because of a severe upper respiratory infection. Harry, now in his 80s, again came into my office, complaining of difficulty in urination and pain in his upper legs. Examination revealed a possible prostatic malignancy, and x-rays confirmed metastatic disease to his bones. He underwent palliative therapy, which temporarily improved the situation. But within a few months it was clear that living alone was becoming difficult for him.

I asked, "Harry, where would you like to go to receive proper care and nourishment? You really are not being fair to yourself living alone. You need help."

"I'd like Leah to take care of me. I could live with my daughter-in-law, Leah, and granddaughter, Jean."

"Have you talked to them about this?"

"No. But I must do that. Don't you think they'd be willing to take care of me?"

"They may be, but I think you should discuss this with your daughter-in-law. If she agrees, I'll be glad to take care of you there."

Harry returned about a week later. He said, "Leah will take care of me. I'm going to move down there next week."

It had been less than a year since her husband had died, but Leah seemed willing to take care of Harry. I thought she probably considered that her late husband would have wanted her to assume this responsibility for the care of his father.

Her terminally ill father-in-law wasn't always the easiest to care for, but she gladly took him into her home. He had a great deal of pain with his problem. She administered to him daily, bathing him, feeding him, cleaning his urinary and fecal mishaps, administering his medications, relieving his pain, and giving him emotional support even though they had never had a close relationship before this final illness. After many months, Harry joined his son, Fred, in death.

Now something unbelievable occurred. Within a few months of Harry's death, Leah received word that his estranged wife, Margaret, had uterine cancer in its terminal stage and wanted to leave California and come home to Lancaster County to die. Who would take care of her? Yes! Leah! Margaret expected Leah to take care of her, so she could come home to be among her sisters and family.

Leah came to the office one day to tell me of this development. She asked me, "Will you look after her medical needs?"

"Yes," I said. I paused. "Do you really want to take care of her?"

"What alternative do I have? None of her sisters is willing or able to take care of her. They are all old and in need of care themselves. She does have a lot of money."

"Will she be giving you any?"

"I don't know. But I'm aware that she was involved in real estate and owns almost a city block of buildings in downtown Los Angeles."

"Well, it certainly is nice of you to do this. Did you know her? When did your late husband last see her?"

"I met her one or two times. I don't believe Fred had seen her for at least 25 years before he died. She didn't come to his funeral. I'll take care of her, if you'll come to see her. I believe she is almost bed-ridden."

When Margaret arrived, Leah called me and asked me to come out to the house within the next few days to see her mother-in-law.

I stopped to see Margaret a few days later. She was sedated and drowsy but was clearly a pleasant woman. She gave me papers from her doctor in California and told me about her problems. She told me that she did not get out of bed.

I examined her, went over her medicine and suggested she continue her medication as the doctor in California had directed. I told Leah how she might take care of her mother-in-law and recommended that she call in a visiting nurse to visit regularly to assist her. After I said "Goodbye" to Margaret and told her how fortunate she was to have an experienced person, Leah, to take care of her, Leah followed me from the room.

As soon as we got out of Margaret's hearing, Leah asked me to sit down. She had a problem. "Just before my mother-in-law got on the plane, some members of a cult she has been friendly with produced some papers and asked her to sign them."

"Did she sign them? What were they?"

"She told me the papers were her will and that she signed all of her estate over to them. What shall I do?"

"I think you should see a lawyer. What have you said to her? Do her sisters know?"

"I really didn't say much to her. I was so shocked when she told me. I did talk to her sisters, and they were upset, too."

"You see a lawyer."

Leah consulted a lawyer about this last-minute change in her mother-in-law's will. He advised her to talk to Margaret's favorite sister about this change in her will; then both of them should talk to her about it.

Later Leah told me that they had had a very nice discussion, and Margaret really did not want to give all of her money to the cult. She claimed that she had been unduly influenced. Members of the cult had pressured her to decide in a few minutes, because her plane was about ready to leave. Margaret suggested that they contact a lawyer, insisting that she would like to change her will and not provide anything for the cult.

Once again, Leah came through. She provided excellent care for her mother-in-law, who was confined to bed and required care for all her needs. I provided medication primarily for pain relief and rest. Leah, in spite of all the cards seemingly stacked against her, continued to give full physical and emotional support to her mother-in-law.

Margaret's lawyer, in the meantime, was working on invalidating her will and making a new one. The lawyer arranged a time at which he, his secretary as a witness, Leah, Margaret and I could all be together for the purpose of writing a new will. We needed to administer her no medication for several hours ahead of this event, so I could truthfully attest to her mental competence and clarity. Margaret and her lawyer discussed the details of the contents of the intended document. After listening to the lawyer read her last will and testament with members of her family as the beneficiaries, Margaret was able to sign her new will in the presence of the witnesses. She died a few weeks later.

For the first time in three years, Leah was left alone with her daughter—and no terminally ill relative to care for. She had done a superb job under stressful and unusual conditions.

I'm happy to report that Margaret did remember Leah in her new will.

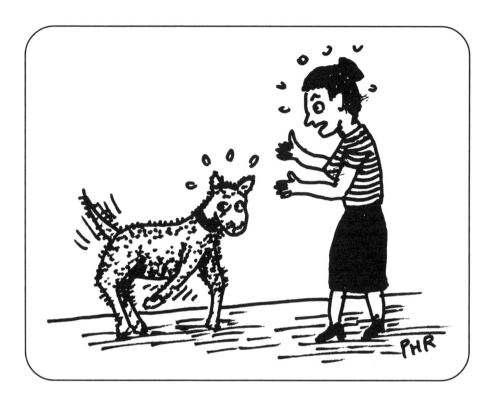

A MAN'S BEST FRIENDS

A DOG AND A NEWSPAPER

One day in the 1950s I was called to a farm because an accident had occurred. I sped through beautiful rural country, past fields of corn and tobacco that had not yet been taken into the barn.

When I arrived at the farm, a woman got into the car beside me and directed me into the field. I inquired, "What happened?"

"I'm not sure," she said, "but I think my husband got his arm in a corn picker."

In a few moments she pointed to her right, "There, you can see Ray's tractor over there. You can drive over that hard path and get to him."

I drove as close as I could to the area of the accident and got out of the car with my bag. As I climbed into the tractor, I could see the farmer's left arm hanging limply over the steering apparatus.

"I'm having a lot of pain in my arm. I think it's broken. Can you give me something to ease the pain?"

Considering how long he must have been sitting there in agony, I agreed that the first thing to do was to give him some relief. "I'll give you this 'shot' first, Ray, and then the pain will start subsiding while I examine you."

"Okay, Doc. I need something quick. It seems like hours since all this happened."

I gave him an injection of morphine. "What happened? Does it hurt here?" as I checked his upper arm and elbow.

"No. It's all below."

His hand was ripped into shreds, with fingers dangling. His lower arm was open, and I could see bone fragments near the surface. I asked his wife, "Please hand my bag up here."

I soon had sterile gauze and bandages at my command. For padding and immobilization I placed thick slabs of gauze on both sides of his hand and started wrapping. I extended this bandaging to his lower arm and soon had his large open wound covered. But I had no splint. Then I spied a newspaper lying beside Ray. Doubling the paper several times I placed his hand and lower arm on this make-do paper splint and started wrapping. I fashioned a sling around his neck and arm, then asked him, "Can you get down on the ground with our help?"

"Sure. I feel better than I've felt for an hour."

His wife and I helped him down. To call an ambulance and await its arrival would take twenty minutes, I estimated. I could get him to the hospital myself in that time. So I said, "Get into my car, and I'll take you to the hospital to get your arm and hand fixed."

After Edith, his wife, and I got Ray into the front seat of my car, I gathered all my equipment. I asked Edith to get in and we drove off across the fields toward their house. "Do you want to go along, Edith?"

"No, let me out at the house. I must tend to some things there and then I'll drive in myself. That way I'll have a car to come home in. Will he be staying in the hospital?"

"Yes. Here we are. Call the hospital, 299-5511, and ask for the emergency room. Tell them we're on our way with a man who has a compound fracture of his lower arm and of his hand. Ask them to have a surgeon there to meet us," I said, as we drove up to the porch in front of the house.

While we were driving to the hospital, I asked Ray, "How are you feeling?"

"The pain has subsided, but I'm upset about my arm and my hand. They must be badly ripped up. Do you think they'll be able to do anything about my hand?"

"I don't know," I said truthfully. "How did you do all of this?"

"I was picking corn and something got stuck. I knew better, but without shutting the motor off I reached inside to unclog it. The worm pulled my arm in, and the only way I could get it out was to rip my caught arm and hand after I turned off the equipment."

"How did you get word to Edith?"

"I always have my dog along, and I sent him up to the house. I was sure they would know there was something wrong if they saw the dog without me."

"You were lucky you didn't have your arm pulled in further."

"I know."

When we arrived at the emergency room I took him in. The surgeon was already there. We explained what had happened. Without further examination, an attendant x-rayed Ray's arm and hand. The operating room was alerted for a "dirty" (unsterile) case, and within a half hour he was being operated upon. I returned to the office as soon as the surgeon took over.

The surgeon called me about Ray as soon as he had finished debriding the wound and treating him. He said, "The arm is broken, and some pieces are missing, but it may heal satisfactorily. I was able to save the thumb and a part of a finger, but the rest is gone and could not be saved.

The next morning I went into the hospital to see several patients. Among them was Ray. When I stopped by his room, he smiled and said, "Look at this." He held out his bandaged limb. "After the doctor fixed my hand and arm, he used the same newspaper splint that you used yesterday in the field. Works just fine, doesn't it?"

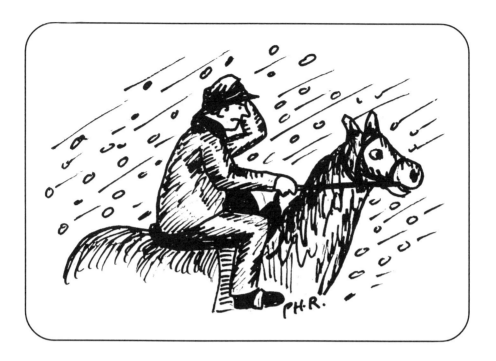

THE LAST LONG RIDE

(The following is based on a conversation I had with Robert L. Bauer, M.D., a country family physician who practiced medicine in Intercourse, Pennsylvania from 1949 to 1967. The story is told in Dr. Bauer's words.)

In February 1958, my wife, Jane, and I had gone to Bermuda for a short vacation.

We flew out of Bermuda at 10 o'clock in the morning to return to New York. We had heard there was a big snowstorm in the Northeast, but we didn't realize until we got over New York City how heavily it was snowing. We circled the airport numerous times. It was one of the few times in my life that I was really concerned, when I looked out the window of the airliner and saw another going in the opposite direction about 100 yards astern of us. We did get down to 200 feet on one approach but were waved off because the runway was covered with snow.

We flew to Norfolk and stayed through one day until 10 p.m., at which time we took off, finally landing at Kennedy Airport about midnight. We now had to find a way to get into the center of New York City, where we were to take a train for Lancaster. The airline was kind enough to charter a bus, because taxi-drivers were charging horrendous amounts to ferry people from the airport to the train terminal.

Finally, we climbed aboard the train about 1:10 a.m. and felt that we were safely on our way to Lancaster.

Shortly after leaving Penn Station, the train stopped. This was to be one of many stops between New York and Lancaster. The snow was so fine that it passed through the filters on the engine and recurringly shorted out the generators. Each time the train had to stop so the crew could clean out the system to get the engine started again.

Eventually, we arrived in Lancaster at about 10 the following morning. It was February 17, 1958. We had been without sleep for more than 24 hours. Jane's mother was at our home in Intercourse with our children. As soon as we arrived at the station, we called home to let her mother know that we had arrived in Lancaster and were all right but tired.

Walking into the parking area of the railroad station, we were able to identify our car only because one green patch of bumper showed through the snow. The railroad provided us with shovels and brooms. We shoveled the car out of the snow and headed for our home in Intercourse, a few miles east of Lancaster. Since we hadn't had anything to eat, we stopped at Joe Myers' Diner, which at that time was in Bridgeport. We knew Joe; and when Jane and I walked into the diner, he said, "Doc, where are you headed?"

"We're going home. We've had no sleep and nothing to eat for the past 24 hours."

Joe's reply was, "You can't get to Intercourse because of the snow." I couldn't understand this, but he went on to explain that it was drifted to the top of the telephone poles in Smoketown. How tall was it? How much snow did we have in Intercourse? Well, Jane's mother, who lived with us, was just five feet tall, and the snowdrift in front of Eli Stoltzfus' Saddle Shop in Intercourse was so high that she could stand on top of the crust and touch the top of a telephone pole. That's proof of the height of the snowdrifts on Newport Road in Intercourse.

After we had eaten our breakfast at the diner, Joe Myers said, "Why don't you go to my house and get some rest?" We readily did so.

We had been in bed about five minutes when the phone rang. It was Jane's mother, who told us that Sadie Fisher, who lived in Georgetown, was in labor. Sadie had just called, she went on, and what did I want to do about this? After I had made the decision to go to Sadie's assistance, I needed to do some planning. First, I needed the proper clothing, then a means of transportation, and finally the equipment to deliver a baby.

Joe Myers, a great hunter, offered his hunting outfit. Now Joe was a short, chunky man, probably about five feet, eight inches tall and weighed 250 pounds and I was six feet tall and weighed 175 pounds. We were of considerably different configuration! My friend, Dr. Henry Wentz, lived in Strasburg and I felt sure that I could get that far. So I called him, explained the situation, and asked him if he had an obstetrics bag that I could use. I had already learned that an Amish man, who had been contacted through a neighbor, would bring two horses into Strasburg; one he would ride, the other was for me.

Without delay we drove to Henry's and Mary's house. Henry handed me his obstetrics bag. I climbed aboard the waiting horse, and the Amish man and I rode out of Strasburg side by side.

At the bifurcation of Routes 896 and 741 at the eastern end of Strasburg, we took Route 896. After we had ridden about half a mile, the Amish man turned into his farm. There was I, astride my horse on the road to Georgetown, with six long, snowy miles to go from Strasburg.

As I left the village, I could see that the wind had caused a lot of drifting. Some places absolutely no snow was on the road; in other areas, the snow would be eight to ten feet deep. So in riding down Route 896, I found it necessary to go around these hillocks of snow.

No vehicle had traversed this road. I was the first. A pioneer on a horse. All alone. Some places I rode through fields because the drifts on the road were so deep.

Fortunately, I had ridden many times before, so I felt quite at home on the horse—but not too comfortable in this cold, windy, snow-covered and drifted environment.

I had hung Dr. Wentz's obstetrics bag on the saddlehorn as I rode. About two miles down the road toward Georgetown, the bag's handle broke. From that time on, it was necessary for me to ride with one hand on the reins and the other holding the bag.

About four miles down the road I recognized that the horse had reached the limits of her endurance. I nudged her into the lane leading to an Amish farm and tied her in the forebay of the barn. Then I walked up to the house, knocked, and said to the man who came to the door, "I'm Dr. Bauer from Intercourse. I'm on my way to Georgetown to deliver Sadie Fisher." (Sadie was no longer an Amish woman but belonged to a Methodist church.)

The Amish man was quite understanding and helpful. He went to the barn and came out with a horse and a mule. Now this jenny mule was a big animal; she might have been 16-1/2 hands tall, and she had long, long legs. When I compared the horse with the mule, standing alongside one another, it was clear to me that the mule was going to be much more capable and sure-footed than the horse, with its shorter legs. I asked, "Is this an easy-riding mule? Will I have any trouble with her, if I ride her?"

"No, absolutely not. You can ride this mule and she'll be fine."

We transferred the saddle and the bag, I clambered aboard, and off we went.

All along the way I knew that people were aware I was going to visit Sadie, who was in labor, because the folks would open their doors as I rode by and tell me that everything was all right at Sadie's home. There were two nurses with Sadie, and they from time to time were telephoning to the folks along the road.

We had left Strasburg at 2:30 p.m. It was now getting dark, and I suppose it was 6:30 or a little later when I arrived in Georgetown. At the outskirts of the town, we came upon a patch of ice on the road. The mule started to skitter across the ice, and down she went. I had one foot on each side of her when she fell but managed to slip off her back as she slid out from under me.

I got the mule back on her feet. Then, with the doctor bag in one hand and the reins in the other, I got onto her back. I rode another half mile from the edge of Georgetown to the Fisher house, which was a one-story bungalow. Next to her home was a more conventional older house with a barn, and that's where I stabled the mule.

Sadie was indeed in labor. When I examined her, I remember that her cervix was probably about six centimeters dilated. The nurses, who had been with her all day long, were there. About 9:30 p.m. a little girl was born to Sadie.

Suddenly, I realized how fatigued I was! Not only had I been without sleep for 40 hours, but also I had ridden six miles through the snow to get to Sadie. The Methodist pastor in Georgetown stopped by and insisted on talking to me deep into the night. At 11 o'clock I'd had as much as I could take. I told him it was time for him to leave. I was going to bed. The Fishers, understanding of my need, provided a bed for me.

The next morning the husband and new father, Harry, was up early. He prepared breakfast for me.

Interestingly, Sadie's probably was one of the last involuntary home deliveries in Lancaster County, though there are even today women, especially among the Amish, who voluntarily deliver at home in Lancaster County.

At a later date, a helicopter from the Middletown Air Force Base flew into Georgetown and took out another young woman who had gone into labor. From that time on, pregnant women in Lancaster County who would be unable to be attended by a physician or midwife in such circumstances, were transported to the hospital by helicopter—at that time by Air Force helicopters and today by private services.

Following breakfast, and after making sure the baby and mother were doing well, I got on the old jenny mule, rode her back, and left her at the farm where I had borrowed her. I transferred the saddle to the horse left there and continued my ride toward Strasburg. I remember seeing the first robin of the year along the side of the road among some bushes next to a farmhouse. What a welcome sight that bird was in the middle of all the snow!

The Amish man came and took his horse home. My wife, Jane, had spent the night with Henry and Mary in Strasburg. How happy we were to get in our car and return to our home in Intercourse to see our children and Jane's mother. It was an exciting end to a wonderful vacation!

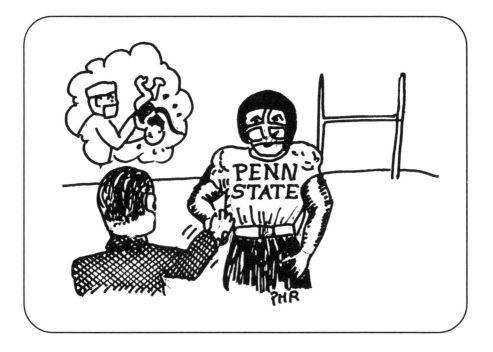

FROM BABY TO
FOOTBALL HERO

The phone rang.

"Is this Dr. Wentz?"

"Yes."

"This is Dolly Hostetler. We received some extra football tickets to Penn State football games. We'd like you and your wife to go along to one this year. Which one would you like?"

Without any hesitation I replied, "The Pitt game." That was the beginning of a most unusual day for my wife, Mary, and me.

More than 20 years earlier the Norman Hostetler family had moved to our area. While living here for two years, they had a baby, Ronald, whom I had had the privilege of delivering into this world. Ronald and his younger brother, Douglas, were now football players at Pennsylvania State University.

Mary and I had some reluctance about traveling to this event. But we both enjoyed football, and seeing the Pitt-Penn State game was a thrill at any time. I had taken care of the Hostetler family many years ago; but what would a big strapping football player care now about the physician who delivered him? And what would any-body in the family care about the doctor's wife?

I remembered the young family quite well. Norman and Dolly Hostetler were Mennonites. During the Korean conflict they had come to our area on "volunteer service" because of their pacifist religious beliefs, as an alternative to serving in the armed forces.

Several other young Mennonite women who were good friends of the Hostetler family were patients of mine. They kept me informed from time to time about the Hostetlers' activities. When two of the boys had made the Penn State football squad, their families went to several of the games.

On one occasion Erma, one of the young friends, said to me, "Dolly says they would like to see you sometime."

I half jokingly replied, "The best place would be at a Penn State football game."

Nonetheless, I was surprised to get the phone call. My wife kept saying, "We'll feel out of place there. After all, the boys and their parents will have friends there. We won't fit in very well."

I suggested, "Let's go and enjoy it. It will be a new experience for both of us, and it could be exciting."

On a chilly, raw Friday night in November we busied ourselves gathering blankets, ear muffs, gloves, hats, scarves, sweaters, and even galoshes—because snow was a probability for the next day.

Early the next morning, we were packed in the car, leaving for Pittsburgh at daybreak on a cold blustery day. We were to meet the Hostetlers at the Pennsylvania Turnpike exit at Somerset, then follow them to the stadium.

At the interchange wc waited only a short time before the Hostetlers arrived. Dolly got into the car with us and we joined a caravan of four other cars on our way to Pitt Stadium.

As we approached an exit off the interstate highway to go into Pittsburgh, traffic slowed to a crawl and sometimes a standstill. At times I wondered if we would get there in time for the beginning of the game. But as we struggled along going through alleys and back streets, we finally drove in sight of the stadium.

The next obstacle was to find a parking place. We lucked out there, too, as we sighted a place a few blocks from the stadium.

As we got out of our car and walked toward the arena, we were bundled up and carrying blankets and warm ski caps. The Hostetlers had brought snacks, hot soup, coffee and tea. We had wonderful seats with the families of the players. It was cold and began to snow and blow. My feet were saying, "We're freezing. Can't you keep us warm?"

But what a football game! Penn State won. Ronald Hostetler, the defensive captain, was the hero and was given the game ball. He had made significant tackles and intercepted and deflected several passes in his role as middle linebacker. We met the coach, Joe Paterno, and the team physician and other players. Then they held a news conference.

When we were finally ready to depart the stadium, it was snowing hard. We were going to the Hostetler home in Hollsopple, near Johnstown. With my wife and me in the car were Dolly and her husband, Norman; Ronald, their son, and Ronald's girl friend. Ronald gave me directions as I drove over roads unfamiliar to me. As the snow increased, my vision of the road decreased. Eventually, I relinquished the driving to Ronald. On the way to the game we had asked Mrs. Hostetler questions about the boys and their activities. Since we were now all together, Dolly said, "Why don't you ask Ron the questions you were asking me? You can hear what he has to say."

"How do you react to being a football hero?" I asked.

"Hero? In our family you don't get to revel in that state very long. My kid sister says, 'You aren't so big. You don't even know how to fix the car when it doesn't run,' and my father says, 'Don't let your head get too big. It won't fit in our family.' My friends and family keep my feet on the ground."

"How did you pick Penn State?"

"I was thinking about other schools but I always wanted to go to Penn State under Paterno."

"Your mother says that Joe Namath called you."

"Oh, did she tell you that story? Yes, one day I was working around the house and my mother called, 'Joe Namath is on the phone. He wants to talk to you.' I answered the phone and the voice on the other end said, 'I'm Joe Namath.' 'Yeah,' I said, 'who is this really?' He said, 'I'm Joe Namath. I'm calling to talk to you about going to the University of Alabama to play football.' After he talked for several minutes about all the advantages I would have at Alabama, I gave him my answer: 'I'm going to Penn State. I don't care for your lifestyle.'"

When we arrived at the Hostetler home, it was all alight, and the warmth inside was not just from the fireplace. It was the genuine warmth of love and friendship. The tables and counters were piled high with food of all kinds. There were salad fixings, sandwiches and entrees just waiting to be served. Dolly had gotten things ready before she had left in the morning, and neighbors had helped before we arrived. But first, after all the guests had arrived, we had a prayer of thanksgiving for the game, the food, and the fellowship. This was followed by hymns of praise to the honor and glory of God and the Savior, Jesus Christ.

A festival of eating followed. We met Doug and their younger brother, Jeff, who was playing quarterback on his high school team at that time—and who would later star as a West Virginia quarterback as well as the quarterback of the New York Giants and the Oakland Raiders. We met other members of the family as well as friends and neighbors. There was an abundance of good fellowship along with the delicious food. Nobody, young or old, felt isolated or out of place. We heard many of the goals and aspirations of the young people who were with us.

Dolly said, "Now Ron, I want you to come over here in front of the fireplace and have your picture taken with Dr. and Mrs. Wentz. This is the doctor, who delivered you."

Ron replied, "Sure! How did you enjoy the game, Dr. Wentz?"

"It was a great game and you played so well. I'm proud of you. You made several key tackles and intercepted or knocked down a couple of important passes."

We continued talking as others took photographs of us.

After a great Christian celebration, with full stomachs and warm hearts, we departed for home in the cold and the dark. "Did you feel comfortable during this experience?" I asked.

Mary responded, "Comfortable! I never so much enjoyed an event that I had looked forward to with such apprehension. After all, you knew the parents and delivered the baby. I didn't know a soul until today. What warmth! What friendship! Ron even had his picture taken with the doctor who delivered him. And what a feast, and everything was so good! Certainly this was a different celebration of a football victory than I had ever experienced."

The long, snowy drive home was shortened and warmed by our conversation and fond memories.

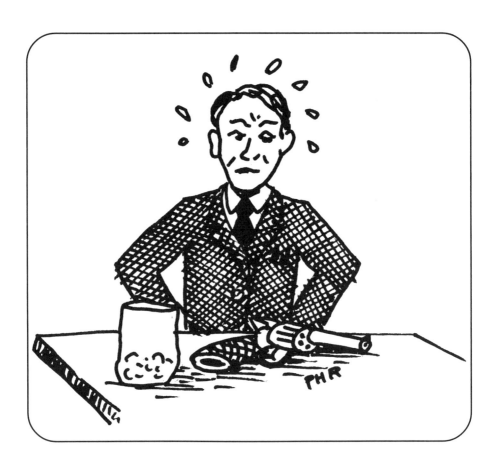

THE GUN WAS LOADED

I was on weekend call for our five-physician group at Eastbrook Family Health Center, situated a few hundred feet off Route 896 just north of Route 30.

It had been a busy day. The traffic, mostly tourists, was horrendous. So instead of spending time on the highway going to my home in Strasburg (about three miles to the south), I had decided to stay in the office and watch a football game on television between seeing patients. On this Sunday, a beautiful autumn day was coming to a close. As the darkness gathered, I sat alone in the library at the front of the building intent on the game.

I thought I heard a sound. I had left the front door unlocked so that anybody seeking medical help could walk in. I walked out of the library into the hall, leaving the television set on. "Hello."

I was a little startled when I heard a voice in return say, "I have a bag of pills in one hand and a gun in the other."

SILENCE!

All kinds of thoughts raced through my mind. Was this a hold-up? How much money was in the office? Was it somebody after drugs? What would happen if I turned on the lights to see who was here? I thought, "What do I have to lose by putting some light on the problem?"

I flicked the switch. The light revealed a bearded man in his 30s. He was wearing an open sport shirt and jeans. Bedraggled, tired. Managing to regain my voice, I asked, "What can I do for you?"

"I've walked 10 miles or more, all the way from Quarryville, with these pills and a gun. I'm trying to figure out which way to end it all, and here I am."

I switched on the light in my personal office and invited him in. I said, "What are your problems? Tell me about them."

He laid the pills and gun on my desk, then blurted out, "Don't touch that gun. It's loaded!"

As I hastened to reassure him that I wouldn't, he seemed relieved to finally stop his wanderings and to find somebody who would listen. He began, "My wife left me and took my daughter with her. I would have shot myself but I can't. I love my daughter too much. I want to see her again."

"What problems did you have with your wife?"

"We've had problems for a long time. We fight constantly. She spends too much money and doesn't keep the house clean and is always running around. I still love her, though."

"Have you had any counseling?"

"No. I just want to see my daughter, Jane." I listened as he continued to list the many faults he found in his wife.

"What are you willing to do about your problems?"

"At this point I'm willing to do almost anything. I want to see my daughter."

"Are you willing to go to the hospital?" I asked. "You really need a lot of help. The first thing we must do is protect you from yourself until you feel better about things. Then we can help you to resolve some of these problems."

"Yes. I've reached the point where I'm willing to do anything to get some help. I can't go on like this."

"Which hospital would you prefer?"

"The General, I guess."

"You wait here while I call a doctor and get permission for you to be admitted. May I take the gun and pills and put them in a safe place while we are making arrangements?"

I looked around my office to see whether anything was lying around with which he could harm himself. When I left the office, I took a letter opener and scissors with me, along with the pills and gun, breathing a sigh of relief that I at least had the gun out of his reach.

I needed to call a psychiatrist for permission for this man—by this time I'd learned that his name was Harold—to be admitted to the hospital. I'd also urged that precautions against suicide be taken. While I awaited the return call from the physician, I asked Harold whom I should call to take him to the hospital. After all, I was so relieved that he was cooperative. I didn't want anything to upset him.

"I'd like my brother-in-law, my wife's brother, Jim, to take me in. And tell him to bring along my daughter. I want to see her. But I don't want to see my wife."

"Where can I reach him?"

He gave me a Quarryville telephone number to call. Jim answered and I gave him implicit instructions: "Bring his daughter. Do not bring his wife! Harold is willing to go to the hospital for some help." Jim assured me he would come in about half an hour with the daughter.

Shortly thereafter the psychiatrist called. I told him the story, and he approved Harold's admission and told me he would see him in the hospital later that evening. I said, "I'm unfamiliar with guns. I don't even know how to unload a gun. The office will be full of employees and patients tomorrow, and I certainly don't want a loaded gun around."

He said, "After the patient leaves, call the police. They'll take care of it for you." I would be alone with the patient until Jim and Jane arrived.

We chatted about his daughter, his 10-mile walk, the weather, his wife, his brother-in-law and various experiences of his life until his transportation arrived.

His brother-in-law entered my office with Jane, the daughter, along with an adult woman in her late 20's. I assumed she must be the brother-in-law's wife. Then I saw the expression on Harold's face. He had run to embrace his daughter, ignoring the adult woman. She was inquiring, "What's wrong, Harold?" and I realized that this woman was his wife!

I really had not secured the loaded gun very well. In all the turmoil I was so anxious to get it away from Harold that I had been quite satisfied at the moment to have put all the potential weapons in the reception area, not expecting any further crisis.

Now I kept one eye on the loaded gun and one on all the participants as best I could, praying that no violence would erupt. When the brother-in-law took him in tow and they all disappeared out of the door, I was relieved. In fact, I had forgotten to tell Jim to which hospital he should go. So I ran out of the door and yelled to them to take him to the emergency room at the Lancaster General Hospital. I said I was calling ahead to let them know he was to be admitted.

I sat down to pull myself together and realized that my job was not done. The loaded gun had to be dealt with. I called the state police barracks, which was only two miles away on Route 30. When I said I had a loaded gun in the office that I wanted to have unloaded, the man on the other end of the line barked, "What are you doing with a loaded gun? Where's the man who brought it to the office? What are you going to do?" When my answers apparently didn't make much sense to him, he said that a policeman would be there shortly.

Within minutes an East Lampeter Township police officer was at the office. He was calm and understanding as I showed him the loaded gun. He said that he was not allowed to unload it for me and started to ask questions: "How did you get the gun? Who brought it in here? Where is he now?" As I tried to explain, he wrote things on a paper and left, saying somebody else would come and unload the gun.

Shortly afterward a state police officer arrived. He asked me what my problem was. I appreciated the depth of protection I would receive if I ever needed it. But at this moment I was overwhelmed with the trouble I was having in trying to get a gun unloaded or trying to give it away. When I started telling my story again, he interrupted with a series of questions: "Where did you get it? To whom does it belong? Why was it brought here? Where is your gun permit? If it isn't yours, where is the person who brought it in?"

I told him, "A patient entered the door about one and a half hours ago with this gun. He had been contemplating suicide. I talked with him, and he consented to go to the hospital for treatment. I only want the gun unloaded or removed."

"What was the patient's name?"

"Harold Minter"

"What's his address?"

"Look, I don't want to get this man in trouble. He has enough trouble. Do you realize he came here for help because he was so depressed he was going to commit suicide? Please unload the gun or take it away."

"You don't understand. It's illegal to have a gun in one's possession without a gun permit. He must be prosecuted, and you must bring charges."

"That cuts it!" I said. I had had enough.

"I will not give you any more information about him. He went to the Lancaster General Hospital to be admitted to the psychiatric unit. If you need more information about him, you can go to the hospital and ask there. This young man is having enough troubles. I'm trying to help him, not harm him. I don't want to bring any charges. I am not interested in increasing his difficulties. My only concern is that I don't know anything about a gun, and this gun needs to be unloaded. A lot of people will be in this office tomorrow, and I don't want anybody to get hurt."

"But it is illegal for you to have a loaded gun," replied the officer.

"You may have the gun. I don't want it."

After a bombardment of questions, which I tried to answer as best I could although at times I felt as if I were a criminal, he left. The loaded gun was still in my possession.

My concern over what to do about the gun didn't last long, because another man soon entered the office. He said, "I'm a gun inspector from Harrisburg. What's going on here?" He began with the same barrage of questions. After I had repeated many of my answers, I said, "Please help me get rid of this gun. That's all I want."

He replied, "I can take care of that" and promptly left taking the gun with him. I felt as if a weight had been lifted from my shoulders.

One day several years later, during regular office hours, I was examining a man who had an upper respiratory infection. When I looked at his chart, I found these words: "Sent to Lancaster General Hospital. Potential suicide attempt by gun or drug overdose. Having marital problems. Cares for daughter very much...."

I realized that he was the same man who had entered the office with the bag of pills and the gun several years previously. Now he was clean-shaven, had a cheerful countenance and was well dressed. As I smiled at him and he returned a smile, I felt a quiet inner satisfaction that his life had changed and that he once again felt in control.

And this time neither of us had a loaded gun!

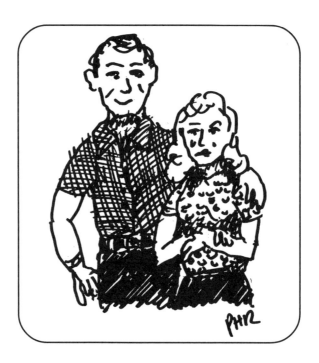

HER FIRST ACCIDENT

The Shoemaker family was one of the first that came to my office when I began my family practice at Strasburg in 1948.

Melvin was about 17 years old, had received a burn across his face and singed his hair. We successfully treated this mishap without any scar or other after-effects. Later, I was able to watch Melvin's life evolve into marriage and children and from farming into other fields of endeavor.

Many years later Melvin brought his oldest daughter, Christine, into the office as an emergency. She was 16 years old, had had a driver's license for a few months, and had been given the family car to drive alone for the first time that evening. Unfortunately, she had had an accident. Her father was called to the scene. Although Christine insisted she was all right and nothing was wrong, her father maintained that she should see a doctor and brought her to see me.

"Were you knocked out? Where do you hurt?"

"It was really a minor accident. I was conscious the whole time. I have this bruise on my arm and another here on my leg. But I'm fine. There's nothing wrong with me."

"Sit up here on the table. Let's check a few of these things."

I examined her head and eyes and pupillary reactions, had her take a deep breath, palpated her spine and examined her chest, abdomen and extremities.

As I was examining the arm and leg that did have slight bruises, Christine said, "I wish everybody had a father like mine. I was dreading his coming. This was the first time I was allowed to drive alone, and this had to happen. I thought he'd be furious. Instead, when he arrived he asked how I was, and then proceeded to comfort me. He put his arms around me and said that it was too bad this happened on my first trip. He told me not to worry, nobody was hurt and everything would be all right. You'll never know how good that made me feel. I feel okay now. May I go?"

Completing my examination, I told her to take aspirin if she had much pain and to apply ice on the bruises to keep down the swelling.

Then I turned to Melvin and said, "She should be all right. You certainly handled this traumatic experience for Christine in a fine way. She will remember your compassion for a long time."

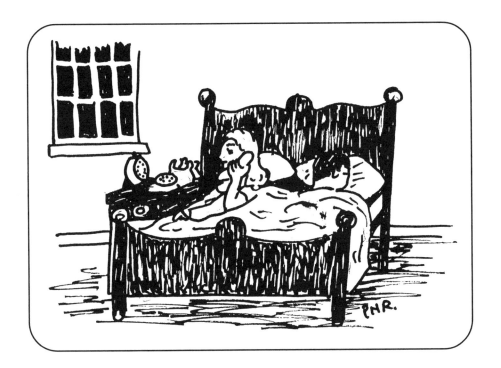

WHO IS THAT MAN
IN BED WITH YOU?

One night I was called to the office to see a man with acute abdominal pain. Cal said, "My stomach hurts so much I can hardly talk." He walked into the office bent over at the waist, holding his abdomen with both hands. He was perspiring and was unable to sit down. He kept pacing the floor holding his belly.

I asked his wife, who had driven him to the office, "How long has he been complaining of his stomach?"

"He awoke with this severe pain about 2 a.m. But really, he has been complaining of his stomach off and on for years. He takes Tums and Maalox by the carload. In the past two weeks I have noticed that he's been chewing on those things more than usual. He has always insisted upon not going to a doctor, so I never could get him to see you."

Cal's abdomen was tense and rigid, and I was unable to isolate any specific area of tenderness. His pulse was 110 beats a minute and his blood pressure was a bit elevated at 152/88. But his heart sounds were good and the rhythm was regular.

I asked his wife about any preceding illnesses, operations or accidents, and she knew of none. Cal interrupted to say, "This is the first time I've seen a doctor since I was a little kid. Aren't you going to give me something for my pain? I can't stand it any longer."

"Yes, right now. I wanted to get a little history and feel your belly before I gave you anything."

I gave him a good dose of a narcotic and asked, "Do you want your wife to take you to the hospital, or should I call an ambulance?"

"My wife brought me over here. She can take me to the hospital. What's wrong?"

"I believe you've had an ulcer in your stomach off and on for years and early this morning it perforated causing your severe abdominal pain. You will need an operation to repair the hole in your stomach. What surgeon do you want me to call?"

"You know the surgeons, Doc. You call the best one. Where shall we go?"

"Go to the emergency room of the Lancaster General Hospital, and I'll have the surgeon meet you there. I'll let the emergency room know you are on your way and will ask them to get some studies done immediately. By the time you get there, you may be a little groggy from the medication. Let the attendants place you on a litter and wheel you into the emergency room."

After they left the office, I called in to inform the emergency room personnel that Cal was on his way and would need some help to be wheeled into their facility.

It was about 4 a.m. by the time I called the surgeon. I knew him and his wife well, so I said to the woman who answered the telephone, "May I speak to the man in bed with you?" Immediately the phone was slammed down, and I was cut off!

Then I started wondering: "Did I call the right number? Was that the surgeon's wife who answered? Should I call back, or should I call another surgeon? If I called the same surgeon immediately and had the right number in the first place, I thought, his wife would know who had placed the first call."

Finally, I called—I think I called—the same number as before. This time a man answered the phone. It was the surgeon I was trying to reach in the first place. I told him about Cal and said he was on his way to the emergency room at that moment. I named the studies I had ordered stat (to be done immediately) and the medication I had given him in the office. He said that he would go in to see him and take care of Cal.

To this day, thirty years later, I don't know whether I called a wrong number first, or whether I called the same number twice and the surgeon answered the second time. Certainly both he and his wife would have been awake, and he may have answered to see who was harassing her!

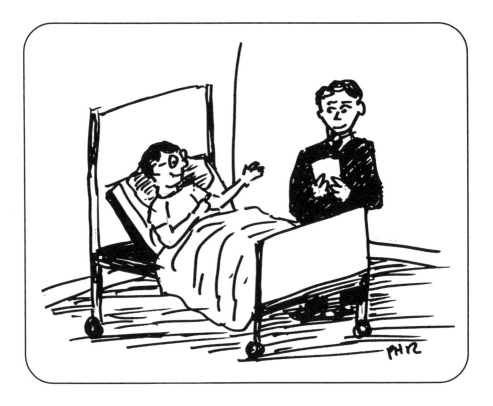

AN INSPIRATION

My wife and I moved into a retirement home at Willow Valley, just south of Lancaster.

Each day the hostess would seat us for dinner with different people. One evening we were seated beside a man in a wheel chair, who was with his wife and sister-in-law. We talked for several minutes before I realized who the man was. It was amazing I should be seated beside him. I didn't even know he was a resident in this retirement village. It brought back memories of an experience I have never forgotten, because Harold Herr has always been an inspiration to me.

In the early 1970s, I was working as the supervisory and teaching physician at the Model Family Practice Unit in Quarryville for the Lancaster General Hospital.

One day a call came in about an emergency in a field along Route 222. One of the family practice residents responded. He went out to find a man with both legs caught in a corn picker. Mr. Herr had been working on his farm, picking corn with this machine. When the corn picker became clogged, he placed a foot in the machine to unjam it. His leg was caught, so he put his other leg into the machine to release the first one. Now both legs were caught in the corn picker!

With help the resident succeeded in removing both crushed and torn legs from the corn picker. He sent the injured man to the hospital in an ambulance. As a result of this horrible accident, Harold Herr lost both of his legs above the knees.

One or two days after the accident, I entered his hospital room to see him. Thinking of the importance of two strong legs to a farmer, I had prepared myself to see an angry man who was depressed and terribly upset. "How are you?" I inquired, apprehensively.

With a smile on his face, Mr. Herr replied, "I'm fine. How are you, Dr. Wentz?"

As we talked, he seemed so cheerful and upbeat I couldn't understand it. After a time, curiosity got the better of me. I asked, "How can you feel so cheerful after this terrible accident?"

"I have a great faith in God, Dr. Wentz. God will take care of me."

After Harold Herr recovered, he continued to run his farm and do most of the work. He never did master the use of two artificial legs, so he walked on his stumps as an abnormally short man.

Now his son manages the farm.

The lesson taught by this man's example has always been an inspiration to me. The attitude he demonstrated was so completely outside my experience with people who were going through a very difficult time.

You can find inspiration in the Bible stories about the faith of Abraham and Noah and Jacob and many others. But here I saw with my own eyes and heard with my own ears the story of a living faith. I had witnessed the faith of Harold Herr that made more of an impression on me than all the stories I had read in the Bible.

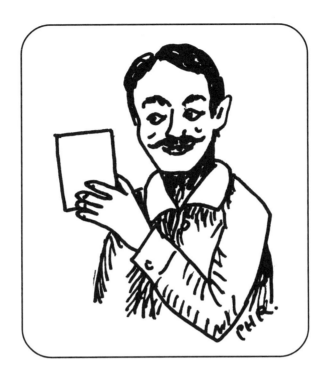

"INSTANT PICTURE"

LEADS TO MEDICAL COOPERATION

Mary and I, together with a dentist, Mark, and his wife, Thelma, went to Honduras to work under Care/Medico. Physicians can help Third World countries in essentially two ways: by treating people, or by helping native physicians treat people. The philosophy of Care/Medico is to help native physicians treat their patients and to provide some medical education along the way.

We stayed in a small hotel at Santa Rosa de Copan, in the western part of Honduras. I worked with Dr. Lopez in a hospital medical ward in which children and adults were thrown together. Honduras' border war with San Salvador had just ended.

I was impressed that each patient, without exception, had some stage of three medical problems: malnutrition, parasites and anemia. The illness that had brought him or her to the hospital, whatever it was, was superimposed on these three underlying medical problems.

In some instances two patients were in the same bed: a child with an adult or two small adults. I saw patients with typhoid fever, measles, dysentery and other infectious diseases as well as patients with heart and lung ailments.

Some children were dying with measles. Patients with severe dehydration were given one liter of intravenous fluids, and antibiotics were being used in small doses. I suggested increasing the amount of fluid given to dehydrated patients and increasing the dose of antibiotics to patients with severe infectious diseases. Within 48 hours, we had consumed all of the intravenous fluids and antibiotics available. That was my first lesson in the Third World.

As soon as Dr. Lopez observed that I was there and could take care of the patients for which he was responsible, he disappeared. So my role as teacher and helper to a native physician appeared short-lived.

As a Lions Club member, I attended the Lions Club meeting in Santa Rosa de Copan. On my arrival I was surprised to learn that the club meeting was being held in the home of Dr. Lopez. The Polaroid camera had just recently made its way to market. I had brought along one of these cameras, with several packs of film. I took several photographs at the Lions Club meeting, and everybody was amazed at the "instant picture." I usually gave the pictures to one of those whom I had photographed. As the meeting and social event drew to a close, I suddenly realized that Dr. Lopez had been in almost every picture. As I thanked him for the fine evening, I suggested, "If you come to work at the hospital tomorrow morning at 9 o'clock, I'll take your picture with your patients."

From then on, he was at work every morning at 9, and we worked together the rest of the month I was there. By the time I left, I had used all of my film and I brought very few pictures home with me, because Dr. Lopez had almost all of them!

In the Third World I learned a lot about treating patients. As a result of a miracle invention, the Polaroid camera, I was able to help a native physician. We communicated well and learned from each other. He taught me about tropical diseases, limiting the quantity of intravenous fluids and the doses of antibiotics to his patients; he emphasized the significance of multiple disease problems in the same patient. I was able to pass on to him the latest techniques and treatment of infectious diseases.

For me it was a valuable and unforgettable experience.

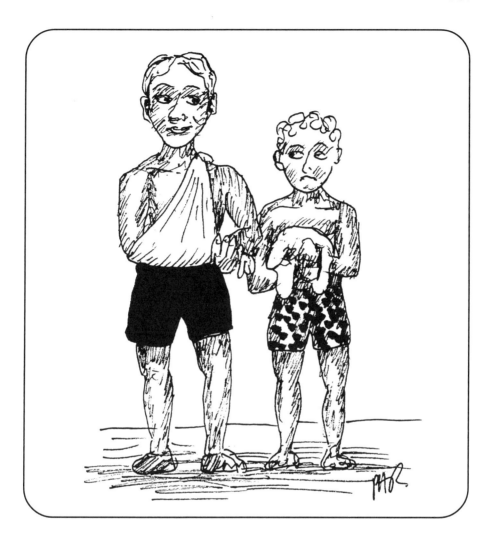

CARING:

THE ONE THING THAT HASN'T CHANGED

As I entered the door to the emergency room of the Lancaster General Hospital, I knew something was wrong. I had my right forearm across my waist, holding it in my left arm although a sling had already been hung around it. The woman behind the counter asked, "What's your problem?"

"I slipped and fell on my right arm. I think it's broken."

"What insurance do you have?" My wife had already gotten out my insurance cards and I passed them over with my left hand.

After she typed the information she needed into the computer, she returned my cards and said, "You may have a seat."

I had been seated less than a minute when I was ushered into the emergency room treatment area. There I met a sympathetic and compassionate man I later learned was a nurse by the name of Robert Doyle. He assisted me onto a litter. Another nurse checked my blood pressure, temperature and pulse.

Bob gently and thoroughly examined my right elbow, shoulder and arm. I had feared that the examination would involve palpation, pressure and motion to see what was wrong. There was gentle palpation, but none of the other. The sling and bandage were gently removed, the area examined and a fresh bandage applied.

As Bob started an intravenous line, he asked, "What did you do?"

"I was playing ball with my seven-year-old grandson, Brandon, around the pool at the Days Inn. The ball bounced out of the pool and I went to get it. It had rolled into a concrete drain. Twenty feet more and the drain would be covered, and I wasn't sure I would be able to retrieve the ball if it rolled that far. So I started to run. I hit a slippery spot and fell onto my right side, landing on my hip and arm.

"My right hip hurt a lot, but I was able to move my leg and get up. I cradled my right arm and walked toward the lifeguard and the manager of the pool. On the way, I called to Brandon to get out of the pool and come with me.

"While the manager phoned my wife, the lifeguard, Dennis, examined my arm. It was bleeding like a spring rain. He put on a bandage and then placed a sling around my arm.

"My wife arrived in about half an hour and brought me to the emergency room. So here I am, still in my bathing suit!"

The emergency room attendant had me slip off my wet bathing trunks and put on a hospital gown. I was asked questions about possible allergies, about my medical and surgical history, and about any medications I was currently taking.

As soon as the emergency room personnel knew I was not allergic to any narcotics, they started flowing morphine into my IV. That made it easier to work around my injured arm.

Bob, the male nurse, seemed able to think of everything at once. He called in the emergency room physician, who asked his own questions and briefly examined me. Then the doctor said, "You need an orthopedist. Who would you like to take care of you?"

In the meantime, Bob Doyle had found the time to return to the waiting room. He told my wife the extent of my injuries, then brought Mary and my grandson into the room to see me. Brandon was so sober, still half-scared and in a shaking voice he inquired, "How do you feel, Granddaddy?" He had been so good at the pool. He sat in a chair beside me; then went to a door to wait for Grandma. He got things for me and carried them for me.

This accident had not been on my agenda for the week-end. I was planning fun with Brandon. Miniature golf, a pizza in the evening, maybe baseball. What else is there?

Dr. Westphal arrived. He expertly and efficiently examined my elbow, forearm and shoulder, then said, "We'll get an x-ray. It appears that you have a compound fracture. Maybe a dislocation."

On a gurney I traveled to the x-ray department. It was necessary for the x-ray technician to get my elbow and arm in the proper position for pictures, and that was the most painful thing I encountered. God bless her—she tried to be as gentle as possible. As she moved my arm again, she said, "I need one more picture. I need to move your arm a little more. Can you raise it a little?" After that ordeal was completed, I returned to the emergency room.

Dr. Westphal came in shortly after reviewing the x-ray results. He said, "You have a bad fracture of the head of the radius and the ulna, with dislocation. We need to take you to the operating room and repair your injury. We'll have you there in half an hour. How do you feel? Any questions?"

"I feel pretty good. Taking the x-ray was the most painful, though the technician tried her best. The male nurse has taken grand care of me and my family. We had planned to go to the New Jersey shore in a week and to Europe in a month. Will I be able to do any of those things, or should we cancel?"

"I think you can do both. You'll be in the hospital for 48 hours for antibiotics, and then you'll go home. You can recuperate at the shore as well as any other place. In a month, I think you'll be able to go to Europe, but you won't be able to carry anything weighing over 10 pounds with your right arm. Wait until we get things fixed up and ask me again. You're going to be all right."

It wasn't long before I heard somebody say, "They're ready for you in the O.R. We won't transfer you to an O.R. litter, so you won't have to be moved until you get to the operating room."

I thought to myself, "Another compassionate maneuver."

I was moved through the hospital corridors and onto an elevator, and then to the operating room.

There somebody complained, "They brought him here on one of those E.R. litters." They asked me to move over as they gently supported my arm.

I heard, "I'm going to make you sleepy...," and that was the last thing I remember until I awoke in a large white room with many litters and many nurses. I tried to get out of my litter, but I was closed in with bars on both sides. A nurse said, "Dr. Wentz, you're all right. Relax. Lie down," as she ran over to calm me. I seemed unable to control my impulse to get out of there.

And then I was whisked to my hospital room and moved over to the bed I'd occupy. Mary and Brandon were there, along with Brandon's parents and his brother, Cameron.

Shortly thereafter, Dr. Westphal arrived. He told me he had placed two screws in the radius to hold it together. He had put a plate around the ulna, had taken some bone chips off the humerus, and had been able to place muscle over the screws and plate. All should be fine, he assured me. Everything was back together again.

I saw many different nurses during my 48-hour hospital stay. All of them were pleasant and considerate and sensitive. I was not accustomed to using my left arm for all of my activities. They helped me bathe at the washstand in my room, kept my arm comfortable, and assisted me with all the procedures I found it difficult to do without a functioning right arm. I was thankful for the pain medication that was available for me and for the antibiotics to prevent infection.

In two days I was ready for discharge. I asked Dr. Tom Westphal, "What about Avalon? What about Europe?"

"I want to see you in the office tomorrow. If everything is satisfactory, you may go to the shore on Saturday. In a month, you should be feeling pretty good and you can go to Europe. You won't be able to carry anything over a few pounds with your right arm. But if you pay somebody to carry your baggage, you'll be able to go."

"I'm paying my wife's way. She can carry my baggage!"

The first night at home, I had fever. My thoughts were, "I have developed an infection. They may have to remove the screws and the plate to get rid of the infection. Then I'll have to start all over again." Actually the fever was still from all the trauma and surgery to my arm. Fortunately, no infection developed.

In the days to come I went through physiotherapy. The therapist, Tim, also was gentle and supportive. Things continued to go well.

Why did I write this story? What is different about my injury or medical problem? The answer is nothing, except that this accident occurred to me. But the care I received—all the emotional support and gentleness and compassion and listening and obtaining answers to my questions—made me realize that the one thing that hasn't changed in medical care is the essential ingredient of caring. And I wanted to share the news about the caring I received. Yes, I was a physician. Prior to this injury I had not known any of those in charge of my medical care and they had not known me.

I also was eager to express the caring theme because in my interviews with older, retired physicians, I had gained the impression that nobody is more critical of the medical care given today than retired doctors. I have only compliments to give, and I wanted to inform all medical personnel, not only the ones responsible for my care, about the value of caring and the appreciation of those who receive it.

I would be remiss not to mention the support I received from my wife and family. Along the way, a seven-year-old boy learned a lot about caring for and helping his disabled grandfather.

Henry S. Wentz, M.D.

Henry S. Wentz, M.D., resided in Lancaster County, Pennsylvania, except for attending Duke University and Jefferson Medical College, and for military service. Dr. Wentz lived and worked among the Amish and Mennonites all of his life. As a teenager, he worked for his family's coal, lumber, and feed business in Leola, and later from 1948 until retirement in 1988, as a family physician in Strasburg and vicinity.

Dr. Wentz also enjoyed the privilege of teaching family medicine to young physicians in the Family Practice Residency Program of the Lancaster General Hospital.

As the years rolled by, Dr. Wentz's desire grew to record some of his experiences during medical training and throughout his forty years of family medicine as medicine that will never be practiced the same again. A special section of this book is included about medical practice among the Amish.

Reading these stories will help you understand why "patients are a virtue." Learning consists not only of reading books, attending lectures and seminars, viewing slides and videotapes, but also of listening to patients and their families.